Evaluating a
Pandemic

Other Titles by the Editor

Foreword by Federico Mayor

Evaluating a
Pandemic

Editor

Charles Pasternak

Oxford International Biomedical Centre, UK

World Scientific

W JERSEY · LONDON · SINGAPORE · BEIJING · SHANGHAI · HONG KONG · TAIPEI · CHENNAI · TOKYO

Published by

World Scientific Publishing Co. Pte. Ltd.

5 Toh Tuck Link, Singapore 596224

USA office: 27 Warren Street, Suite 401-402, Hackensack, NJ 07601

UK office: 57 Shelton Street, Covent Garden, London WC2H 9HE

Library of Congress Cataloging-in-Publication Data
Names: Pasternak, Charles A. (Charles Alexander), editor.
Title: Evaluating a pandemic / editor, Charles Pasternak.
Description: New Jersey : World Scientific, [2024] | Includes bibliographical references and index.
Identifiers: LCCN 2023000303 | ISBN 9789811262814 (hardcover) |
    ISBN 9789811262821 (ebook) | ISBN 9789811262838 (ebook other)
Subjects: MESH: COVID-19--history | Health Policy | Health Care Evaluation Mechanisms |
    History, 21st Century
Classification: LCC RA644.C67 | NLM WC 506 | DDC 362.1962/4144--dc23/eng/20240505
LC record available at https://lccn.loc.gov/2023000303

British Library Cataloguing-in-Publication Data
A catalogue record for this book is available from the British Library.

For any available supplementary material, please visit
https://www.worldscientific.com/worldscibooks/10.1142/13039#t=suppl

Desk Editor: Shaun Tan Yi Jie

Typeset by Stallion Press
Email: enquiries@stallionpress.com

In memory of the millions of people
across the world who died from
the COVID-19 pandemic

Foreword

By Federico Mayor

COVID-19 has been a pandemic of the world we live in, a world with immense human traffic. In the past, epidemics were localised precisely because the spread of the causative pathogen was restricted. COVID-19 has already taught us several lessons for the future. The first is that health security is a priority, and it is always necessary to have the technical and financial elements that allow for adequate prevention.

In the face of any pathophysiological condition, it is necessary to know the background, the scientific and technical possibilities for action, and, progressively importantly, the behaviour of citizens. Health security is a fundamental right.

The question has again been raised as to whether it is possible to claim as a right the freedom not to protect oneself, not to vaccinate oneself and thus to be an active transmitter of a serious pathology, which is especially dangerous for the elderly.

This book by Prof. Charles Pasternak is very useful for dealing effectively with future epidemics. An active and dynamic present is necessary for a better future. It is essential to promote research in general and to take full advantage of physical introspection diagnostic systems, which have greatly accelerated the capacity of predictive, prospective and preventive medicine in recent years. The progressive longevity of the human species, with all that this represents, especially in the case of the neurosciences (neurodegenerative diseases), must be taken into account to promote affordability and access for all patients to the infrastructures required, both for diagnosis and treatment and for scientific research.

It is not possible, when talking about security, to continue to think that military force is the only expression and reference for it (see a new concept of security developed by me in my book *Inventar el futuro* (*Invent the future*), that is now being translated into English. Read the Introduction, in English, here: https://fund-culturadepaz.org/wp-content/uploads/2022/09/INVENTAR-EL-FUTURO-Introduccion-Version-2.pdf). This is a very serious mistake, a very costly mistake that generally causes a lot of pain in terms of human and material losses. By thinking in this way, there is a biased vision and a focus exclusively on the war aspects, leaving many other facets of "human" security completely behind, which is, in any case, what should really matter.

I insist: health security must from now on occupy a prominent place in security. It cannot be the case that territorial security leads to the protection of borders and territories but not of the human beings who inhabit them. Fewer bombs and more firemen. Fewer soldiers and more health workers. A big change is needed for the new era.

The difference between the means dedicated to potential confrontations and those available to deal with recurrent natural disasters (fires, floods, earthquakes, tsunamis, pandemics, etc.) shows that the concept of "security" is still being promoted by the major arms producers (see http://federicomayor-eng.blogspot.com/2016/08/). This is anachronistic and, above all, it is putting humanity as a whole at serious risk and calls for a "security contract".

I never tire of recalling that it is not possible for us to continue to observe the arsenals filled with rockets, bombs, planes, warships, and submarines without raising our voices and saying that there are thousands of human beings who die of hunger every day, who live in conditions of extreme poverty without access to adequate health services, without reacting to this crude reality and the progressive deterioration of the conditions of habitability on Earth. We must act without delay because we are reaching the point of no return on essential issues of intergenerational legacy.

We cannot remain silent any longer. We cannot continue to be impassive spectators of what is happening, because we would become accomplices. The scientific, academic, teaching, artistic, intellectual and creative communities, in short, must be at the forefront of popular mobilisation (see https://aeac.science/pacto2019/). This mobilisation must take place now, with great urgency, to ensure the living conditions of citizens who are no longer manipulated by the omnipotent and omnipresent influence of the "great dominion" (military, financial and energy industries, and the media).

Let us say loud and clear to all those who are now responsible for implementing decisions that transcend borders: a new worldview with new lifestyles cannot be put off. The great personal and collective challenge is to change our way of life. The world is entering a new era. We have many things to preserve for the future and many other things to change decisively. At last, the people. At last, the voice of the people. At last, citizens' power. At last, the word and not force. A culture of peace and non-violence and never again a culture of war.

Let us remember the lessons of the coronavirus to usher in *a new era on a global scale with a different personal and collective behaviour* so that everyone, not just a few, enjoys the dignified life that is their due. We have to remember that we cannot go back to "pre-COVID". We have to keep in mind that the circumstances before the pandemic most likely contributed in some way to the situation as we have had to live it.

A radical change of course is indispensable and urgent, with a total rethink of present strategies. The worst that could happen — and we must be very clear about this — is that post-COVID governance would be the same as pre-COVID, because this would mean that we still lack the rules, structures and mechanisms to ensure the exact fulfilment of the guidelines for conduct that were approved at the UN General Assembly in the autumn of 2015 "to transform the world".

"We must change track," wrote Edgar Morin, almost a centenarian. Indeed, we must change track and lifestyle. How wonderful it would be if this were the offspring of COVID-19! The only answer that must now be offered to pave the way for a new era is a radical change in security, investing considerable human, economic and technical resources in food, education, health, ecology, etc., and, in particular, "humanising" care and information services, *putting people where today there is only technology, and paying great psychological attention to all ages, especially the very young and the elderly*. To this end, thanks to longevity, we can count on an under-utilised treasure: the experience of so many retired people who represent a considerable store of remedies.

Federico Mayor
3rd September 2022

Introduction

By Charles Pasternak

In 2020 I was asked by World Scientific, the publisher of this volume, to write a book as part of their ongoing series of works on COVID-19. I was approached because 'I had written philosophical/analytical books in the past'. But I am no Jefferson (remember US President John F Kennedy's remarks to visiting Nobel Laureates in 1962: 'I think this is the most extraordinary collection of talent, of human knowledge, that has ever been gathered together at the White House, with the possible exception of when Thomas Jefferson dined here — alone'). So I decided instead to edit a volume of contributions by experts, not just in science or medicine, but in anthropology, economics, history, philosophy and psychology as well. That is how *Evaluating a Pandemic* came about. Readers will appreciate that new clinical findings and proposals are published in scientific journals on a weekly basis. The aim of this book is to provide a review of the situation in the time period 2020–2022 and to consider how to react to future epidemics.

The COVID-19 pandemic is the result of infections by a virus. Non-scientific readers may find parts of a recent book by John Brooke [1] useful. Such readers are reminded that viruses are particles of protein and RNA or DNA. Sometimes they are enclosed by a lipid membrane. The COVID virus is such an enveloped RNA virus. Viruses are so small that, unlike bacteria, they cannot be seen under an optical microscope. Only with an electron microscope can the features of a virus be made out. Viruses are inert structures. When they have entered a living cell — a bacterium or a cell inside a plant or an animal — they are able to multiply and exit in order to spread and initiate further infections. The virus causing COVID-19 is a coronavirus, so called because short protein spikes protruding through its lipid membrane resemble the decorations on a crown. The virus is named SARS (severe acute respiratory syndrome)-CoV-2 because it is related, in structure and pathogenic consequence, to the SARS-CoV-1 virus that also originated in Asia and caused a worldwide outbreak during 2002–2004. But that virus's infectivity was low: approximately 800 people died, whereas SARS-CoV-2 has so far claimed around seven million lives.

This volume begins with the source of the SARS-CoV-2 virus. Like SARS-CoV-1, its natural reservoir appears to be in horseshoe bats, with palm civets providing a possible intermediary to infection of humans. A large live animal market in Wuhan has been suggested to be the place where transmission from animal to human occurred in 2019. But this remains controversial. **Angus Dalgleish** considers another possibility, one that has been obscured by an apparent cover-up on the part of the WHO and the countries it represents. Professor Dalgleish's conclusion has recently been vindicated by others, including science author Matt Ridley [2] and public bodies like the US Senate [3]. But bats continue to pose a possible source for a future outbreak of SARS-CoV [4], and global warming may precipitate the jump of a virus from a wild animal to a human [5].

2020 saw the start of an exceptionally rapid production of vaccines against COVID-19. These are of two types: 'classical' vaccines and novel mRNA vaccines. Both induce immunity through the 'spike' protein of SARS-CoV-2. The former use an inactivated viral vector, like an adenovirus, to enter human cells. The latter use the mRNA itself, embedded in special lipid particles to gain entry. AstraZeneca (the only company to sell the vaccine at cost) — in conjunction with Oxford University — in the UK, and Johnson & Johnson in the US, have refined the viral vector approach, as did Russia with its 'Sputnik' vaccine. China's 'Sinopharm' and 'Sinovac' vaccines use inactivated SARS-CoV-2 itself. The Serum Institute of India in Pune manufactures the Oxford-AstraZeneca vaccine on a global scale. Novel mRNA vaccines have been effectively manufactured by Pfizer — in conjunction with BioNTech in Germany — and by the newly established company Moderna (based on the words 'modified' and 'RNA') in the US. These are the main SARS-CoV-2 vaccine manufacturers that have been supplying most of the world, but over

200 other pharmaceutical companies are engaged in this enterprise. **Sean Elias** tells the story of the development of the Oxford-AstraZeneca vaccine. **Hana Hassanin** describes the stages that led from laboratory experiments to introduce mRNA into cells — unrelated to viral infections — to the creation of mRNA vaccines. Millions of lives have probably been saved by vaccination (according to mathematical modelling [6]. But given that concerns have been raised about some of the Pfizer-BioNTech clinical trials and that most vaccines are based on what is likely a highly infectious laboratory construct — see Chapter 1 — such figures are in some doubt).

Drugs, as opposed to vaccines, against virus-induced diseases are few and far between. In the case of immunosuppressed patients infected with SARS-CoV-2, for whom vaccines cannot be used, synthetic drugs or monoclonal antibody treatment are the only answer (though nasal sprays may prove effective [7]). Dexamethasone (a steroid) has been used in hospitalised COVID patients on intensive respiratory support, but its efficacy on the less severely ill is doubtful (see, for example, [8]). Initiating clinical trials of new drugs is difficult because of the paucity of areas of infection (due to the apparent success of vaccines) in which to test the efficacy of a novel drug [9]. So it would be premature to devote a chapter to this topic.

Because infected individuals generally exhibit only mild symptoms, it is extremely important to identify such people and to isolate them in order to prevent the spread of the virus to those at risk of severe disease and death. **Anne Hoppe, Aurelia Vessiere** and **Daniel Bausch** assess the diagnostics that have been successful in this regard and speculate how they may be used in future outbreaks — not just of pandemics caused by viral infections, but of endemic diseases as well.

Countries have reacted to the pandemic in different ways. While Japan and Sweden, for example, each avoided a national lockdown — to obvious economic advantage — the consequences have been very different. The former achieved fewer cases and deaths than other G7 countries [10]. The latter did not [11], despite initial hopes that some form of herd immunity might emerge. **Martha Lincoln** examines the nature of the US's response to the pandemic in terms of its national exceptionalism, particularly in relation to the wearing of masks.

The economic consequences of Sweden's 'light touch' response to COVID-19, as opposed to that in the UK with stringent lockdowns, are compared in a scholarly analysis by **David Meenagh** and **Patrick Minford**. Subsequent waves of new infections reflect the emergence of mutant strains in which an amino acid at a certain position in the viral protein is replaced by another [12]. Some of the mutants, such as the Omicron variants, are more infectious but less virulent. Meenagh and Minford have analysed the effects of three waves of new infections in Sweden and the UK during 2020 and 2021. The rates of infection and resultant deaths have been roughly the same. Yet the decline in GDP has proved to be very different: considerably greater in the UK than in Sweden during the first two waves of infection in each country, while during the third wave Sweden's GDP actually grew by 2.2%, whereas that in the UK still fell by almost 2%.

It is not only the economy that suffers from rigorous lockdowns. In the UK the mantra to 'protect the NHS' (National Health Service) meant that the focus of clinical care was on those infected with coronavirus, while potential cases of heart failure or cancer were not followed up. As Professor Karol Sikora puts it, 'I was called a killer for warning of lockdown harms'. He points out that the present cancer crisis — over 300,000 people on England's cancer waiting list — is 'the predictable consequence of the NHS focusing exclusively on COVID-19' [13]. Another consequence of stringent lockdown has been the downgraded education that schoolchildren and university students received over two important years of their lives. Many schools and universities introduced Zoom lectures and classes in order to limit contact between students and their teachers. But distance learning is no substitute for face-to face contact. Was this necessary? COVID-infected youngsters in general suffer far less deleterious sequelae than the elderly, though rare cases of 'Long COVID' — see below and [14] — are an unfortunate outcome. Others have expressed related views (see, for example, [15]). In fairness to the UK government, its lockdown strategy was comparable to that of most other European nations. It was Sweden that proved to be the — successful — outlier.

Most readers of this volume will have experienced a COVID-19 infection (over 650 million people worldwide). The effects are generally mild, and this aspect is not discussed here. The long-term consequences, however, can be serious in some people. They include cardiovascular [16] and other complications. The appearance of small blood clots that affect the function of particular organs may underlie the symptoms of Long COVID: see [17] and the extensive researches by Douglas Kell and his collaborators [18].

In addition to economic issues, lockdown has had two sociological consequences. The first concerns trust to follow instructions between people and the UK government (in both directions), as well as between different groups of people. As **Stephen Reicher** points out, the rapid spread of the virus through human-human contacts was recognised by March of 2020. Italy initiated lockdown on 9 March. In the UK the government was swayed by its Chief Medical Officer's opinion that people would exhibit 'behavioural fatigue' (failure to follow the rules) if too long a lockdown was imposed. It accordingly delayed lockdown until 23 March. This two-week delay, it has been calculated, cost the country some 43,000 lives.

The second sociological outcome of lockdown is that working from home has proved to have had beneficial as well as adverse consequences. Significant effects on the emotional agility of the workforce in regard to commitment, communication and development have been noted by **Ana Martins** and **Narishaa Shah**. They analyse these matters from the viewpoint of the Internal Audit Unit of the eThekwini Municipality in Durban, Kwa-Zulu Natal, South Africa. The authors suggest that their findings are likely to be relevant to many organisations elsewhere in the world.

Epidemics caused by an infectious agent naturally die out after a certain period, as preventative measures and herd immunity begin to slow down transmission. Most of such diseases, as **AC Grayling** reminds us, are spread by human-human contact through overcrowding and poor hygiene. This is true even of as recent an epidemic as the 1917 'Spanish' Flu (that probably erupted in the state of Kansas in the US). So it is not surprising that in the absence of a vaccine or drug against COVID-19 in 2020, some governments initiated measures to criminalise anyone mixing excessively with others in restaurants and bars, places of worship and sporting events. Even two years later, by which time most people in high-income countries had been vaccinated, anyone testing positive was required to self-isolate for a short period (though this was considerably less than the 40 days — *quaranta giorni*, hence quarantine — imposed by the Doge when the bubonic plague hit Venice in 1348 [19]).

Niall Ferguson, another historian, analysed the probable outcome of the pandemic in October of 2020 [20]. Two years on, he shows here how he underestimated some consequences (the effectiveness of vaccines on the one hand, and the overall death toll on the other), while other factors (the initial

xvi   *Evaluating a Pandemic*

success in controlling the outbreak in certain Asian countries like Taiwan and of course China) he did not predict. Nor did he anticipate the resistance towards vaccines, the wearing of masks and other measures in the US, that Martha Lincoln in this volume refers to as that country's 'exceptionalism'.

Naturally occurring pandemics may not pose as big a risk to humanity as the impact of a giant asteroid, but their potential effect on the viability of a large percentage of the population is undoubted. The Black Death (whose causative microbe has been around for more than 5,000 years [21]) killed between a quarter and a half of the entire population of Europe during the 14th century. COVID-19 has proved not to be of that scale, and is therefore unlikely to result in some resistance to the offending microbe [22]. Advances in tackling communicable diseases over the past century have undoubtedly helped to reduce the impact of pandemics. The extent to which COVID-19 is nevertheless posing a global catastrophic risk is discussed by **Tom Hobson, Lara Mani, Catherine Rhodes**, and **Lalitha Sundaram**.

This book contains 11 chapters (said to be a lucky number in Feng Shui). The contributors are all respected academics — there is no active politician or popular journalist among them. Yet I very much hope that such people will read the work. For as Professor Sarah Gilbert (the scientist responsible for creating the Oxford-AstraZeneca vaccine and co-author of one of the best scientific page-turners I have read [23]) said in her 2021 Richard Dimbleby Memorial Lecture, 'We cannot allow a situation where we have gone through all we have gone through, and then find that the enormous economic losses we have sustained mean that there is still no funding for pandemic preparedness. The advances we have made, and the knowledge we have gained, must not be lost.' A similar plea has been made by philanthropist Bill Gates [24]. And as this book was going to press, the science journal *Nature* published a series of short articles on just this topic [25]. But in fact the pandemic is not over yet [26].

I am grateful to John Brooke, Angus Dalgleish, Sean Elias, Martin Rees and Peter Piot for advice, and to Shaun Tan Yi Jie, my editor at World Scientific, for commissioning this volume and for seeing it successfully through to publication.

Readers who wish to make substantial comments, including scientific or clinical data, about any of the chapters are invited to submit these to the

Publisher (Shaun Tan Yi Jie, yjtan@wspc.com) for potential inclusion in a possible 2nd edition.

References

[1] Brooke, J (2022). *Understanding Epidemics.* Austin Macauley.

[2] Ridley, M (2022, September 18). The Lancet Commission is the latest to highlight how seeking the truth has come second to other considerations. *The Telegraph.* https://www.telegraph.co.uk/news/2022/09/18/search-covid-19s-origins-continues-hindered-fear-offending-china/; Ridley, M (2023, February 15). The World Health Organisation is putting us all in danger. The failure to speedily investigate Covid's real origins leave us vulnerable to another pandemic. *The Telegraph.* https://www.telegraph.co.uk/news/2023/02/15/world-health-organisation-putting-us-danger/.

[3] Senate Committee on Health Education, Labor and Pensions. (2022, October). An Analysis of the Origins of the COVID-19 Pandemic: Interim Report. *United States Senate.* https://www.help.senate.gov/imo/media/doc/report_an_analysis_of_the_origins_of_covid-19_102722.pdf.

[4] Mallapaty, S (2022). Tens of thousands of people exposed to bat coronaviruses a year. *Nature,* **608,** 457–458.

[5] Carlson, CJ, *et al.* (2022). Climate change increases cross-species viral transmission risk. *Nature,* **607,** 555–562.

[6] Watson, O, *et al.* (2022). Global impact of the first year of COVID-19 vaccination: a mathematical modelling study. *Lancet,* **22,** 1293–1302.

[7] Kozlov, M (2022). Could a nose spray a day keep Covid away? *Nature,* **611,** 209.

[8] Crothers, C, *et al.* (2022). Dexamethasone in hospitalised COVID-19 patients not on intensive respiratory support. *European Respiratory Journal,* **60,** 2102532.

[9] Sidik, SM (2022). New Covid drugs face delays as trials grow more difficult. *Nature,* **606,** 637.

[10] Oshitani, H (2022). COVID lessons from Japan: clear messaging is key. *Nature,* **605,** 589.

[11] Brusselaers, N, *et al.* (2022). Evaluation of science advice during the COVID-19 epidemic in Sweden. *Humanities and Social Sciences Communications,* **9,** 91.

[12] Calloway, E (2022). Chronic Covid: the evolving story. *Nature,* **606,** 452–455.

[13] Sikora, K (2022, August 12). I was called a killer for warning of lockdown harms. *The Telegraph.* https://www.telegraph.co.uk/news/2022/08/12/called-killer-warning-lockdown-harms/.

[14] Bangham, C (2021, February 19). What do we know about Long Covid? *The Royal Society.* https://royalsociety.org/blog/2021/02/what-do-we-know-about-long-covid/?gclid=EAIaIQobChMI9LH806Hu-QIVFuDtCh3ktg_9EAAYAiAAEgIMQfD_BwE.

[15] Giubilini, A, *et al.* (2022). A focussed protection vaccination strategy: why we should not target children with COVID-19 vaccination policies. *Journal of Medical Ethics*, **47**(8), 565–566.

[16] Sidik, SM (2022). Heart disease after Covid: what the data say. *Nature*, **608**, 26–28.

[17] Willyard, C (2022). The mystery in micro-clots. *Nature*, **608**, 662–664.

[18] http://dbkgroup.org/publications/.

[19] Sobel, D (1999). *Galileo's Daughter*. Fourth Estate, p. 210.

[20] Ferguson, N (2021). *Doom: The Politics of Catastrophe*. Penguin Press.

[21] Ancient DNA shows plague afflicted Bronze Age Crete. (2022). *Nature*, **608**, 243.

[22] Enard, D (2022). Rapid natural selection during the Black Death. *Nature*, **611**, 237–238.

[23] Gilbert, S & Green, C (2021). *Vaxxers: The Inside Story of the Oxford AstraZeneca Vaccine and the Race Against the Virus*. Hodder & Stoughton.

[24] Gates, B (2022). *How to Prevent the Next Pandemic*. Allen Lane/Knopf.

[25] Pandemic preparedness. (2022). *Nature*, **610**, S33–S50.

[26] No room for COVID complacency in 2023. (2023). *Nature*, **613**, 7.

About the Editor

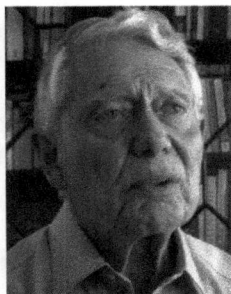

Professor Charles Pasternak is a British biochemist and founding Director of the Oxford International Biomedical Centre, of which he is currently President. He has published over 250 original papers and reviews, and is the founding Editor-in-Chief of *Bioscience Reports*, helming the journal for 28 years. He is also the editor of *Biosciences 2000* (World Scientific, 1999), and author of nine other books.

Educated at Oxford University, Charles Pasternak spent 15 years on the staff of the Oxford Biochemistry Department, during which time he also held a teaching Fellowship at Worcester College, Oxford. He spent two years as a Post-Doctoral Fellow in the Pharmacology Department of Yale University Medical School, and subsequently held an Eleanor Roosevelt Fellowship of the International Union Against Cancer in the Department of Neurosciences at the University of California San Diego Medical School in La Jolla. In 1976 he was invited to move to St George's Hospital Medical School, University of London, in order to set up a new Department of Biochemistry, which he subsequently expanded into a larger Department of Cellular and Molecular Sciences as founder-Chairman. He is currently President of the Oxford International Biomedical Centre, which he founded in 1992.

Charles Pasternak is a tireless promoter of international scientific collaboration. He has been a member of the Executive Committee for a UNESCO initiative on Molecular and Cellular Biology, a member of the Education Committee of the International Union of Biochemistry and Molecular Biology (IUBMB), a member of the International Advisory Board for the Chulabhorn

Research Institute, Bangkok and a member of the Scientific Board of Antenna Technologie, Geneva. In 1979 he founded the Cell Surface Research Fund in order to foster international research links and scientific meetings on various aspects of fundamental and clinical research on the cell surface. In 1993 he received the degree of Doctor Honoris Causa and Palade medal from the University of Bucharest, in 1995 the honour of Amigo de Venezuela from the Fundacion Venezuela Positiva, and in 2002 was elected Foreign Member of the Polish Academy of Arts and Sciences.

About the Contributors
(in alphabetical order of last name)

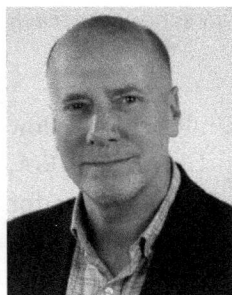

Daniel **Bausch**, MD, is Professor of Tropical Medicine at the London School of Hygiene and Tropical Medicine, UK, and Senior Director of Emerging Threats and Global Health Security at FIND, the global alliance for diagnostics, Switzerland. He is a Fellow, and the current President, of the American Society of Tropical Medicine and Hygiene. He is an internationally recognised leader in global health and emerging diseases, with over 25 years' experience in sub-Saharan Africa, Latin America, and Asia combating viruses such as Ebola, Lassa, hantavirus, and SARS coronaviruses.

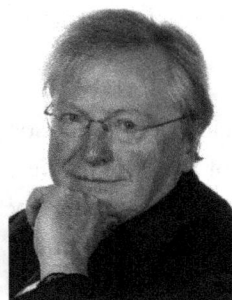

Angus **Dalgleish**, MD, is Foundation Professor of Oncology at St George's University of London, UK, and Principal of the Institute of Cancer Vaccines and Immunotherapy, UK. He is a Fellow of the UK Academy of Medical Sciences, Royal College of Physicians, Royal College of Pathologists, and Royal Australasian College of Physicians. He is best known for his seminal contributions relating to the virology of HIV, and has co-edited five medical books. He is currently interested in the immunology of cancer, especially as applied to melanoma, prostate, pancreatic, gliomas and other solid tumour types.

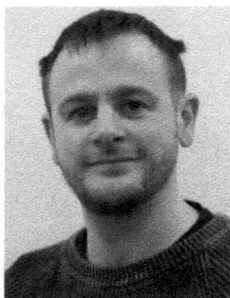

Sean **Elias**, PhD, is Public Engagement Lead in Professor Dame Sarah Gilbert's group at the newly formed Pandemic Sciences Institute, University of Oxford, UK. Formerly of the Jenner Institute, University of Oxford, he has been working in the field of vaccine research since 2008 and was part of the Oxford COVID-19 vaccine development team. During the pandemic he switched from the laboratory to a science communication role, providing science consultation to journalists and news outlets to ensure publications representing the work of the Institute were of the highest quality and were scientifically accurate. Since then, his role has expanded to also focus on school outreach and engagement.

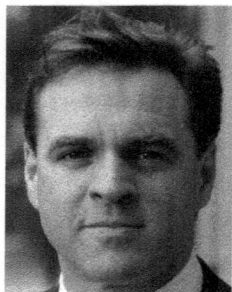

Niall **Ferguson**, PhD, is Milbank Family Senior Fellow at the Hoover Institution, Stanford University, USA, and Senior Faculty Fellow at the Belfer Center for Science and International Affairs, Harvard University, USA. He is a Fellow of the Royal Society of Edinburgh. He is regarded as one of the world's foremost historians, and was listed in *Time* magazine's 100 most influential people in the world in 2004. He has won many prizes for his writing, and of his international bestselling books, the PBS adaptation of *The Ascent of Money* clinched the International Emmy award for Best Documentary.

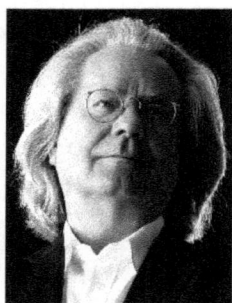

AC **Grayling**, PhD, is Founder, Principal, and Professor of Philosophy at the New College of the Humanities, Northeastern University, UK, and a Supernumerary Fellow of St Anne's College, Oxford. He was appointed Commander of the Order of the British Empire (CBE) in the 2017 New Year Honours for services to philosophy. He is a Fellow of the Royal Society of Literature and the Royal Society of Arts. His main academic interests lie in epistemology, metaphysics, and philosophical logic and he has published over 30 books in these and related subjects.

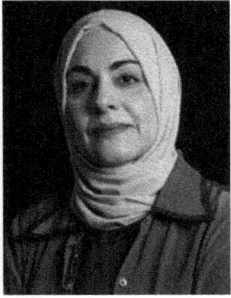

Hana **Hassanin**, MD, is Associate Professor in Translational and Experimental Medicine at the University of Surrey, UK, where she is also Medical Director of the Surrey Clinical Research Facility and Clinical Consultant for the Dementia Research Institute at the Surrey Sleep Research Centre. She has a joint appointment with the Royal Surrey Foundation Trust as the Medical Director of the NIHR Royal Surrey Clinical Research Facility. She is a lead expert in conducting clinical trials and has led over 60 high-scale and complex clinical trials — including multinational trials — in various therapeutic areas both early and late phase covering osteoporosis, vaccines and infectious diseases, cardiovascular, respiratory, oncology, and immunology.

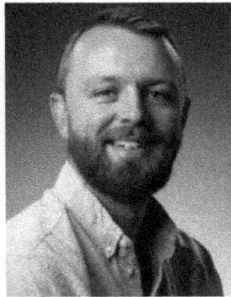

Tom **Hobson**, PhD, is Research Associate at the Centre for the Study of Existential Risk, University of Cambridge, UK, and an Affiliate of the BioRISC initiative at St Catharine's College. His research is concerned with understanding how expert communities and policy actors imagine the future, how present and historical sociotechnical contexts shape their visions of the future, and how they endeavour to secure a particular vision of the future through technology and innovation. Empirically, his work centres on the governance of emerging technologies, biotechnology and biosecurity. He also conducts research on the politics of existential risk and the sociotechnical construction of extreme risks as a category.

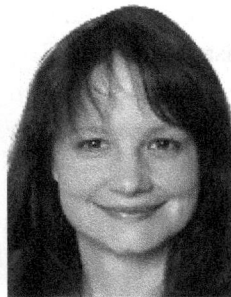

Anne **Hoppe**, PhD, is Director of Innovation at the Elizabeth Glaser Paediatric AIDS Foundation. She leads the Innovation and New Technologies team in identifying promising innovations, developing strategies for introduction of these innovations, and implementing projects to introduce and catalyse scale of beneficial innovations. She has 14 years of experience in directing large-scale infectious disease projects in low- and middle-income countries, with a focus on sub-Saharan Africa; for instance, she built capacity for clinical trials management in Zambia and Uganda.

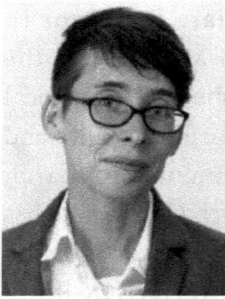

Martha **Lincoln**, PhD, is Associate Professor at the Department of Anthropology, San Francisco State University, USA. Broadly, her research addresses the cultural politics of public health, biopolitics, and the effects of political economic change on health systems and health outcomes. She previously specialized in cultural and medical anthropology of Vietnam, publishing the book *Epidemic Politics in Contemporary Vietnam: Public Health and the State*. She is currently studying affective economies in medical crowdfunding for cancer.

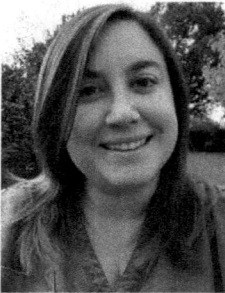

Lara **Mani**, PhD, is Senior Research Associate at the Centre for the Study of Existential Risk, University of Cambridge, UK, where her research seeks to understand the efficacy of various communication methods and strategies for gaining traction for the mitigation and prevention of global catastrophic risks. This research to date has adopted the use of role-playing games for increasing awareness for the importance of AI safety and ethics, and scenario-based exercises for exploring possible futures in biosecurity.

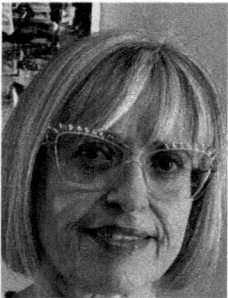

Ana **Martins**, PhD, is Professor of Leadership and Information Science, and was the Interim Dean and Head of the Graduate School of Business and Leadership, University of KwaZulu-Natal, South Africa. Her current research interests embrace emerging concerns for humanising organisations and leadership. Her publications cover topics related to shared and distributed leadership, developing human capital, nurturing spiritual and emotional capitals, trust and tacit knowledge; harnessing communities of practice, social capital, innovation and creativity in teams; development of soft skills; as well as knowledge management and culture.

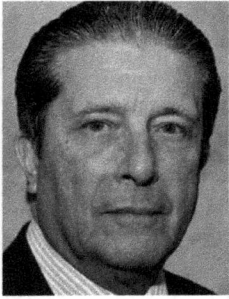

Federico **Mayor**, PhD, is a former Director-General of UNESCO. Originally a Professor of Biochemistry, he became Rector of the University of Granada and Co-Founder of the Spanish National Research Council. In 1987, he was elected Director-General of UNESCO, serving two six-year terms. Under his leadership, UNESCO developed a Culture of Peace Programme that outlined a plan of action addressing education for peace, human rights, and democracy, ending poverty, cultural diversity, and conflict prevention and resolution. In 1999, he returned to Spain and started the Foundation for a Culture of Peace (Fundación Cultura de Paz), of which he is currently President.

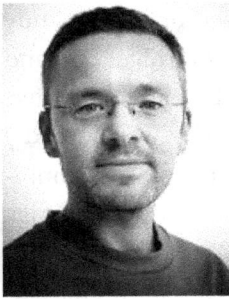

David **Meenagh**, PhD, is a Reader in Economics at Cardiff Business School, UK. His research focuses on applied macroeconomics, with the main aim to improve macroeconomic modelling methods in order to better inform macroeconomic policy.

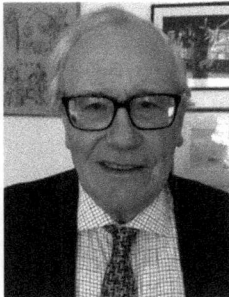

Patrick **Minford**, PhD, is Professor of Applied Economics at Cardiff Business School, UK, where he is also Director of the Julian Hodge Institute of Applied Macroeconomics. He was appointed Commander of the Order of the British Empire (CBE) in the 1996 New Year Honours for services to economics. His main research interest is in macroeconomic modelling, and his Liverpool Model was influential in forecasting and policy analysis during the 1980s. He rose to prominence in 1981 when 364 leading economists published a statement criticising Margaret Thatcher's economic policies, and Thatcher named him as one of two economics professors who supported her strategy.

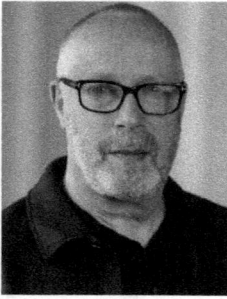

Stephen **Reicher**, PhD, is the Bishop Wardlaw Professor of Social Psychology at the University of St Andrews, UK. He is a Fellow of the British Academy, the Academy of Social Sciences, and the Royal Society of Edinburgh (of which he is also Vice-President). His research is in the area of social psychology and group behaviour. More specifically, he attempts to develop a model of crowd action that accounts for both social determination and social change, construct social categories through language and action, and understand political rhetoric and mass mobilisation — especially around the issue of national identity.

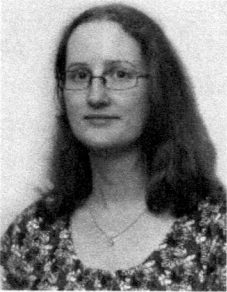

Catherine **Rhodes**, PhD, is Research Affiliate (formerly Executive Director) of the Centre for the Study of Existential Risk, University of Cambridge, UK, and Research Affiliate at the Biosecurity Research Initiative, St Catharine's College, Cambridge. Her work broadly focuses on understanding the intersection and combination of risk stemming from technologies and risk stemming from governance (or lack of it). She has particular expertise in international governance of biotechnology, biosecurity and broader biological risk management issues.

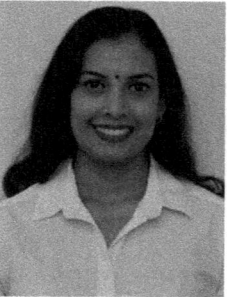

Narishaa **Shah**, MBA, is a Continuous Security Audit Specialist at eThekwini Municipality based in Durban, KwaZulu-Natal, South Africa. Her work focuses on audit reviews in terms of "Security" within the municipality. She is also currently studying for her Doctorate at the Graduate School of Business and Leadership, University of KwaZulu-Natal. Her study interest is focused towards transcending human consciousness in the workplace, which aims to nurture individuals in understanding themselves first as a basis for developing new business growth and knowledge.

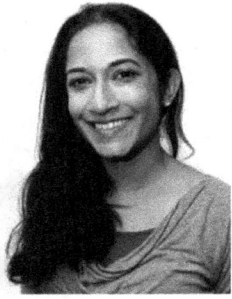

Lalitha **Sundaram**, PhD, is Senior Research Associate at the Centre for the Study of Existential Risk, University of Cambridge, UK and an affiliate of the BioRISC initiative at St Catharine's College, Cambridge. Her research is in the area of bio-risk, with a particular emphasis on regulation and governance. She investigates risks — real or perceived — surrounding emerging biotechnologies such as synthetic biology.

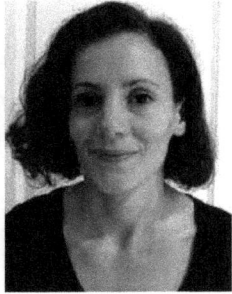

Aurélia **Vessière**, PhD, is Deputy Director of Pandemic Threats Programme at FIND, the global alliance for diagnostics, Switzerland, where she addresses gaps in the availability and use of diagnostic tests for pandemic preparedness and response. Trained in virology and epidemiology, with specialisation in tropical infectious diseases, she has more than 15 years of experience in sub-Saharan Africa engaging in clinical research, diagnosis and epidemiology of emerging viruses, as well as HIV, malaria and tuberculosis.

Contents

https://doi.org/10.1142/9789811262821_0001

Chapter

1

The Origin of the COVID-19 Virus

By Angus Dalgleish

Summary

Analysis of the published sequence of SARS-CoV-2 from an early patient with COVID shows the presence of a short sequence of amino acids in the spike protein that is absent in samples taken from nine different horseshoe bats. This lends credence to the proposal that COVID-19 was not passed to humans directly from an animal in the Wuhan live food market. Rather it is likely that the virus escaped from a laboratory where it was being modified to make it more infective and hence a better source for a vaccine.

Introduction

It is more than three years since COVID-19 appeared in Wuhan, Hubei, China, and subsequently swept around the world, yet there is no consensus on the origin of the virus and how the pandemic started. The first official account of the illness that appeared in the Western press is attributed to a young ophthalmologist who warned his colleagues in late December 2019 that a mysterious viral infection was killing people in Wuhan. He noted that the disorder was very infectious and causing respiratory symptoms similar to those reported in the SARS epidemic of 2002–3. SARS stands for Severe Acute Respiratory Syndrome and SARS-CoV-1, as it is now known, was a coronavirus which was subsequently shown to have originated in bats and jumped to humans via an intermediary host, probably a masked palm civet, a racoon dog or a Chinese ferret badger [1]. The doctor, Li Wenliang, who recorded his observations on an online chat room in order to warn his colleagues, was reprimanded and told to deny his report by the local police. This event was subsequently reported in the *New York Times* (6th February 2020) after Dr Li died of the very disease about which he had tried to warn the world. The first official report of the infection came from Dr Zhang Jixian, a respiratory specialist with experience of SARS-CoV-1 years before, and who was working at the Hubei Provincial Hospital. She had noticed an atypical pneumonia presenting with highly unusual lung changes on CT scanning. Cases within the same family suggested it was highly infectious and likely to be a virus. Dr Fen, Director of the Emergency Department at the Wuhan Central Hospital, had also seen a similar case and tests indicated it was likely to be a SARS coronavirus. These cases, when reported to the Wuhan Health Commission, resulted in an instruction to the hospitals not to make anything public. This resulted in leaked notices online, which eventually alerted the Chinese Centre for Disease Control and Prevention (CDC) Director, Dr George Gao, who on contacting the Wuhan Disease Control Office was informed that several cases (at least 27) had been occurring since the beginning of December (reviewed in detail by Chan & Ridley) [2].

The world did not learn of the outbreak until the end of December when Dr Marjorie Pollock, Deputy Editor of ProMED-mail, the largest public global surveillance system monitoring infectious disease outbreaks, became aware of the foregoing from internet posts. A cluster of cases had been in contact with the Huanan Seafood Market and this was rapidly shut down and cleaned with disinfectant. Even after this action, doctors were accused by hospitals of 'spreading rumours'. It was nearly three weeks of suppressing data that confirmed human-to-human transmission before the authorities admitted that the virus was being spread in such a manner on January 20th, 2020 (reviewed in detail by PR Goddard) [3].

The seafood market was suspected as the cause of the spread and this was presented as the case for several months, even though many patients had presented with no links whatsoever to the market. Eventually the Chinese authorities admitted that there was no evidence that the virus originated from there. In the meantime, valuable datasets describing early COVID-19 cases had been deleted from databases, leading to the observation by Dr Jesse Bloom of the Fred Hutchinson Cancer Research Centre that there was a less than wholehearted effort to trace the source of the epidemic [2].

The virus, taken from a patient sample on December 26th, 2019, was first sequenced by Zhang Yongzhen of the Shanghai Public Health Clinical Centre. The sequence was uploaded to the GenBank database run by the National Centre for Biotechnology Information in the United States. It was, however, to be embargoed until July 2020. The paper was submitted to *Nature* [4]. A co-author, Dr Holmes, who had not previously seen the full sequence, persuaded Dr Zhang to share it, and the latter obliged and uploaded it on virological.org. Dr Zhang suffered a 'crackdown' by the Chinese National Health Commission, who told all laboratories to destroy all COVID-19 samples or transfer them to designated institutions. Dr Zhang had his laboratory completely shut down. The sequence of the virus revealed that it was indeed a coronavirus, with similarities to SARS and was thus designated SARS-CoV-2. It was assumed that it had a high probability of coming from a zoonotic source as the sequence was similar to a bat coronavirus.

As news of the outbreak leaked out, the Chinese authorities had initially told the WHO that the disease was completely under control and that human-to-human transmission was impossible. Yet Chinese media had reported many cases as early as November 2019, and the virus may have started to infect people even earlier than that. As the scale of the outbreak became apparent, the Chinese authorities accepted that the virus was indeed spreading through human contacts. All city-to-city travel was immediately stopped, but the Wuhan International Airport was surprisingly left open. The only railway left in operation was from Wuhan to the airport. As hundreds of flights a day to Europe and the US took off, the virus naturally spread to the rest of the world.

The WHO did not initially consider the outbreak as serious. They had been very critical of the way China had handled the SARS-CoV-1 epidemic in 2003. The WHO director at the time, Gro Harlem Brundtland, had been censorious of the way it had been managed, but China seemed to have considered the WHO to be the problem rather than its own management. A possible scenario is that the Chinese subsequently set out to acquire greater influence within the WHO. They achieved this by lobbying for a more compliant WHO head, Dr Tedros Adhanom Ghebreyesus from Ethiopia, to take over from Dr Margaret Chang in 2017. This weakening of the WHO probably played a major role in the disastrous spread of the epidemic as countries were completely unprepared, having been assured by the old WHO team that a future outbreak of a SARS-like disease could be rapidly contained and would never become established beyond Asia.

Now We Have a Virus, Where Did It Come From?

SARS-CoV-1 and the Middle East Respiratory Syndrome (MERS) had clearly come from animals, with the civet being cited as an intermediator for SARS, and the camel for MERS. The origin of SARS-CoV-2, however, is clearly linked to coronaviruses from bats. The original occurrence of COVID in Wuhan was surprising as the only link with bats was with its virology institute. The fact that COVID was associated with a virus with similarities to SARS-CoV-1 and other bat coronaviruses was the main reason why the origin of SARS-CoV-2 was assumed to come from bats with or without an intermediary species. The Wuhan Institute of Virology (WIV) had a particular interest in bats and had been searching for SARS-like viruses since the first SARS outbreak. The team was led by Dr Shi Zhengli, Director of its Centre for Emerging Infectious Diseases, who was christened 'Bat Woman' by the world's media. Dr Shi and her group sampled thousands of bats in the wild and took swabs and blood samples to examine in her laboratory. They sequenced the viral genomes and studied the interaction between the viruses and cells. They also altered some genomes in order to better understand their biology and to see whether they could become human pathogens. Dr Shi focused on caves in southern China where the bats lived [5].

An important event in this story is the episode of an outbreak in 2012 of respiratory symptoms in miners working in the Mojiang mine of Yunnan province in southwest China. They had been working on clearing the former copper mine of guano, which is used as a fertiliser as well as a component in traditional Chinese medicines. Six workers were admitted to hospital and two of them died. The serum from the survivors was sent to the WIV and found to be positive for SARS virus antibodies [6]. It is worth noting that the 2012 incident came to light only in 2020 when an anonymous Twitter user called 'the seeker' unearthed a medical thesis by a student, Li Xu, on "The analysis of 6 patients with severe pneumonia caused by unknown viruses". It concluded that the virus was a SARS-related coronavirus and that it was essential to investigate the bats further [6].

Dr Shi did discover a novel SARS-like coronavirus and published a part of its sequence in 2016 [5]. It was from a different species of bat to the ones known to harbour the progenitors of SARS: *Rhinolophus affinis*, an intermediate horseshoe bat, rather than *Rhinolophus sinicus*, the rufous horseshoe bat. What was surprising was that a further eight SARS-like viruses were discovered (but not mentioned until 2020) and no link was made between the new sequence published in 2016 and the disease which had killed workers in the mine in 2012. The intense research and discussion regarding the virus from the mines did lead to Dr Shi's group publishing an addendum to the original sequence [7, 8].

SARS-CoV-2

Dr Shi established that the new virus isolated from Wuhan COVID patients had a 79.6% match with the SARS-CoV-1 virus of 2002–3. However, another group had noticed a 98.9% match with a fragment of the 2016 virus (named 4991) and Dr Shi's group confirmed a 96% genome match with a sample from a *Rhinolophus affinis* bat in Yunnan. SARS-CoV-2 was accordingly the name given to the causative agent of COVID-19. The sequence from the *Rhinolophus affinis* bat was named as RaTG13 and had no previous citation. It was later added to the Chinese database when it was spotted to have 100% identity to the 2016 published variant 4991 that had been isolated from the mine in 2012 [5, 7, 8].

This history reveals that much important data had been withheld and that the virus which caused COVID-19 clearly was associated with bats and animals associated with the meat market.

The basic facts of the origin of COVID-19 are that it is not only *similar* to SARS-CoV-1, which came from bats, but is *identical* to the fragment obtained from the agent that was associated with the illness developed in the mine workers in 2012 that was being analysed in the WIV laboratory. No other virus reviewed by Dr Shi's team had this sequence. The virus involved was only found in bats living 1,800 km away from Wuhan and which had been brought to the WIV for further study.

Evidence Against a Zoonotic Infection Becomes Available But is Ignored

For a virus to jump species often requires an intermediate reservoir host to which it becomes adapted, with multiple attempts, with mutations and Darwinian selection for viruses that can more easily infect the host. It is possible that it could jump directly to humans but it is noteworthy that SARS-CoV-1 came from a civet cat or racoon dog and MERS from a camel. These intermediate hosts were identified within 4–10 months. So far, no such host for SARS-CoV-2 has been found.

The sequence of the circulating virus suggests that its origin may be the horseshoe bat *Rhinolophus affinis*. This, however, is only found in the Yunnan province (over 1,800 km away from Wuhan). Moreover, three different laboratories have reported that the virus can no longer infect bat cells, which means at the very least that an intermediate should be found [9]. As 40% of the initial patients worked or shopped at the seafood market in Wuhan, this suggested one of the animals there as a possible source. However, the animals present in the market during the likely zoonotic transfer were not tested. These animals included racoon dogs, a species known to be susceptible to infection with bat-like SARS viruses [1]. Whilst it is possible that zoonotic transfers occurred within the market, it does not explain how the virus got there in the first place. So the 'ultimate' source of the virus is bats but the proximal source in the market is unknown, as all the animals tested were found to be negative for evidence of SARS-CoV-2 antibodies, and hence it would therefore be more likely to be from the WIV.

As previously mentioned, zoonoses occur when the conditions are met and may take several months, with different mutations occurring at random, whilst the virus jumps from the animal to humans. In the case of SARS-COV-1 there is evidence of a gradual evolution. Thus the pre-epidemic spike protein had fewer than 30% of all the changes it would later develop by the time it achieved human-to-human spread and became an epidemic. This explains why SARS-CoV-1 and MERS could be detected in archived human blood collected pre-epidemic in 0.6% of specimens [9]. In the case of SARS-CoV-2 there is absolutely no evidence of such a footprint of a pre-pandemic infection in either humans or animals.

What the most surprising outcome of the whole history of this pandemic is that everyone from the original scientist to scientific advisors and politicians, as well as editors of learned journals and the mainstream media, accepted that the origin was a natural jump from a bat or other animal. The emerging evidence for such a zoonotic jump remained completely negative. No bat-infected animals in the Wuhan Animal Market were found and no serological evidence for a slow evolving presence prior to the first Wuhan cases has been found anywhere. Not only was the evidence that a natural origin could not be supported by any evidence to date ignored, but the paradigm that it was natural was hammered home in high-profile papers, discussed below.

We now know that suspicions were aroused very early on by those who had access to the first sequences that the virus had some highly unexpected features. Nevertheless, via the Freedom of Information Act it was revealed that Dr Anthony Fauci, Director of the National Institute of Allergy and Infectious Diseases (NIAID) in the US and Chief Medical Advisor to the President of the United States, took the lead in suppressing any discussion that it may not be a natural virus. This appears to have been accepted by Sir Patrick Vallance, Chief Scientific Officer of the UK, as well as by Sir Jeremy Farrar, the Director of the Wellcome Trust, apparently on a joint telephone call. Furthermore, it would appear that Fauci encouraged coronavirus experts such as Kristian Andersen to write a paper to *Nature* arguing that SARS-Cov-2 could not be other than a natural virus [10]. Dr Fauci then seemed to have used this paper to 'prove' that it had a natural cause. However, this paper by Kristian Andersen and colleagues alerted many to features more akin to non-natural viruses by citing references to viruses which came from laboratory manipulations.

Another high profile attempt to 'cement' the natural origin theory was by Peter Daszak and colleagues who published a statement in *The Lancet* in support of scientists, and Chinese scientists in particular, claiming that any suggestions that the virus may have leaked from the laboratory were conspiracy theories to be ignored [11]. All signatories claimed to have no conflict of interest, yet all but one were associated with the EcoHealth Alliance (EHA) organisation of which Peter Daszak was the head.

The EHA paper drew attention to the fact that the EHA had received grants from the NIAID, whose head is Dr Anthony Fauci. The EHA funded bat coronavirus work in Dr Shi's lab, which included genetic manipulation to enhance the ability of bat viruses to infect human cells. This work included a collaboration with Dr Ralph Baric at Chapel Hill in North Carolina, who is a world expert at splicing RNA without leaving a trace. These two papers were written by authors the vast majority of whom were all involved in genetic manipulation of biological organisms [10, 11].

The narrative up to now was that COVID-19 had to have a natural origin and that the only alternative, that is manipulation in the laboratory and then leakage, was impossible as the WIV was impenetrable with regard to biosafety.

Evidence that Laboratory Virus Leaks do Occur

There are four levels of biosecurity for laboratories, the safest being BSL-4, reserved for the most lethal viruses, such as Ebola and Lassa Fever. SARS viruses require BSL-3 conditions. It is important to realise that the Foot and Mouth agent escaped from a BSL-4 facility and that SARS has already escaped on at least six occasions and infected people in Singapore (2003), in Taiwan (2003) and four times in Beijing (2004). The Beijing incidents resulted in transmission and symptoms in the contacts of the lab worker, including a nurse who was hospitalised. The denial of the possibility of a laboratory leak is strange, considering the fact that a 2018 inspection of the Wuhan labs had been very critical of safety issues, and it is unlikely that all SARS experiments were conducted in BSL-3 facilities [2].

Even if the most stringent precautions are taken, dangerous pathogens can still leak out and cause pandemics and/or kill humans. The Pirbright leak of Foot and Mouth Disease, which caused seven million cattle to be slaughtered, was not due to poor operating procedures but due to a leaking drainage pipe outside the immediate laboratory [12]. Moreover, the last death from smallpox was a lab photographer who worked two floors down from the research laboratory in which smallpox was being handled. She was infected via the joint ventilation system. The head of the laboratory committed suicide over his responsibility for death [3].

Could a Virus from a Laboratory in the Wuhan Institute of Virology Have Escaped and Caused the Pandemic?

SARS-CoV-2 seems to have been almost perfectly adapted to human cells from the very beginning. This adaption could not have happened in a seronegative community, otherwise there would be evidence of previous infections, leaving an antibody trace. On balance it seems that the evidence for a zoonotic leap, which everyone agreed was the most likely origin, completely lacks any data to support it. It is possible that the virus was not completely adapted to human infection in the laboratory and/or underwent gain of function (GOF) experiments without necessarily being capable of person-to-person spread. Some zoonotic transfer may have taken place in the market but it is extremely unlikely to have originated from it. It is, however, possible that some combination of many things (passage in human mammalian cells, GOF modifications, zoonosis) resulted in such an odd SARS virus.

The Wuhan Institute of Virology

The WIV is one of the leading coronavirus research institutions in the world. They are documented as having thousands of virus specimens in their possession and at least 300 characterised viruses from bats. These were on a public website until September 2019 when they were removed. Without any hint of irony, the reason given was to prevent it from being hacked.

When Dr Shi and colleagues finally published the SARS-CoV-2 sequence in *Nature* they discussed various features of the genome but failed to mention the presence of the 'elephant in the room', namely the Furin Cleavage Site (FCS) which is not present in any other coronavirus of the same subgenera [13]. The importance of this is that the spike protein, which attaches to the ACE-2 receptor on human cells, requires a host enzyme called Furin to activate it at a spot on the S1/S2 junction. Other viruses in this clade of coronaviruses do not have this and are cleaved at another site further downstream, known as S2. This was most peculiar as Dr Shi had previously published on successfully adding it to a bat coronavirus. A separate Wuhan laboratory had also published that they could create a FCS in a coronavirus [14, 15].

Gain of Function Research

The very fact that GOF research was being performed in the WIV is extremely important and not even a secret as many papers have been published showing how inserts can enhance activity of coronaviruses [14–16]. Indeed, adding a

FCS, first performed on SARS-CoV-1, has been performed in many laboratories, including the WIV. Following this realisation that SARS-CoV-2 has a FCS, numerous papers, mainly from Chinese labs [17], tried to show how the FCS could have been naturally acquired from distant cousins of SARS-CoV-2. This might have been through recombination between two different viruses that have infected the same host, copied their genetic material and swapped sequences. However, natural viruses that do have FCS insertions are in animal hosts that do not exist in the Hubei province.

Detailed Analysis of the Published Sequences for SARS-CoV-2

With the publication of the sequence in *Nature* there was a 'race' to take the 'spike' protein containing the receptor binding domain (RBD) and insert it into a number of delivery systems in order to create vaccine candidates.

My colleague Birger Sørensen in Oslo, Norway had developed a highly unique and effective HIV therapeutic vaccine, called Vacc-4X. Unlike all the main failed vaccine candidates developed since the HIV virus was first sequenced, it did not use the whole envelope (with its RBD for CD4 receptor). Here we both agreed that vaccines should be defined by omitting everything except the most important epitopes, which will not vary from isolate to isolate. Birger had chosen just four epitopes for his HIV vaccine, which was effective in a phase II randomised trial [18].

Analysis of the spike protein using blast analysis revealed that 78% of the spike protein had human homology and therefore should be omitted from any vaccine candidate because of reported severe side effects [19, 20]. This detail has been ignored by nearly all published 'COVID' vaccine candidates to date [21]. It was chosen because it would induce antibodies to the RBD, which had been shown to bind to the main cell receptor, known as ACE-2, and present on many cells involved in controlling cardiovascular function and blood pressure in particular. It is relevant that many GOF experiments had used human ACE-2 receptors in cell lines to optimise coronavirus infection [22, 23].

However, whilst determining what the core epitopes were to use in our proposed non-full spike vaccine candidate, it became evident that this virus had other unusual features other than the FCS already mentioned.

The main unexpected discovery was that the surrounding non-RBD contained highly charged 'inserts' incorporating unusual amino acid substitutions. This means that the extra positive charge can allow interaction with non-ACE-2 receptors, such as the C-type lectin tail on the CD209L/L-SIGN and CD209/DC-SIGN receptors [30]. These receptors are known to enable endocytosis into the cells by other highly pathogenic viruses. In addition, the 'spike' protein has a very high charge with an isoelectric point of 8.24, compared with only 5.67 for the 2003 SARS spike protein (Figures 1.1 and 1.2). Together these charges enable SARS-CoV-2 to bypass the ACE-2 receptor by making salt/arginine bridges to infect non-ACE-2 bearing cells. This property may explain many of the highly unusual features of COVID-19 infection, such as the loss of taste and smell, which suggests direct invasion of the taste and smell bitter/sweet receptors. They are known to be associated with innate immune system function and may precipitate further infection of other cells. Early attempts to publish these data and warn others not to use

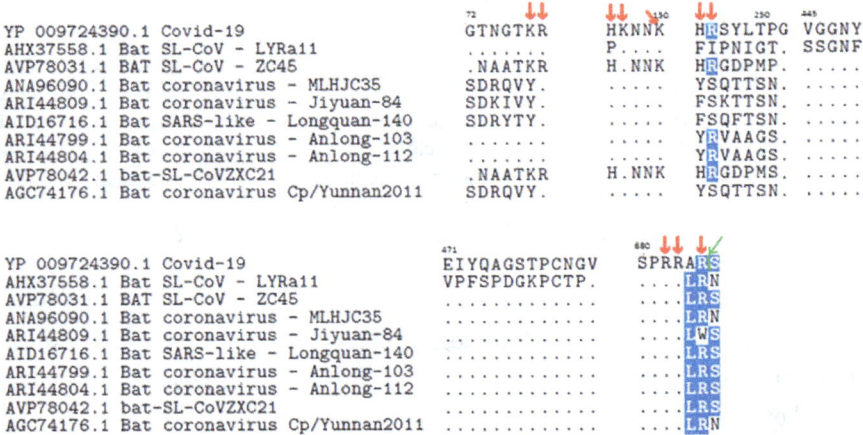

```
                                               72    ⬇⬇     ⬇⬇ ↘150   ⬇⬇    230   445
YP 009724390.1 Covid-19                      GTNGTKR  HKNNK  HRSYLTPG  VGGNY
AHX37558.1 Bat SL-CoV - LYRa11               .......  P....  FIPNIGT.  SSGNF
AVP78031.1 BAT SL-CoV - ZC45                 .NAATKR  H.NNK  HRGDPMP.  .....
ANA96090.1 Bat coronavirus - MLHJC35         SDRQVY.  .....  YSQTTSN.  .....
ARI44809.1 Bat coronavirus - Jiyuan-84       SDKIVY.  .....  FSKTTSN.  .....
AID16716.1 Bat SARS-like - Longquan-140      SDRYTY.  .....  FSQFTSN.  .....
ARI44799.1 Bat coronavirus - Anlong-103      .......  .....  YRVAAGS.  .....
ARI44804.1 Bat coronavirus - Anlong-112      .......  .....  YRVAAGS.  .....
AVP78042.1 bat-SL-CoVZXC21                   .NAATKR  H.NNK  HRGDPMS.  .....
AGC74176.1 Bat coronavirus Cp/Yunnan2011     SDRQVY.  .....  YSQTTSN.  .....
```

```
                                             471               680 ⬇⬇ ⬇✓
YP 009724390.1 Covid-19                      EIYQAGSTPCNGV  SPRRARS
AHX37558.1 Bat SL-CoV - LYRa11               VPFSPDGKPCTP.  ....LRN
AVP78031.1 BAT SL-CoV - ZC45                 ............   ....LRS
ANA96090.1 Bat coronavirus - MLHJC35         ............   ....LRN
ARI44809.1 Bat coronavirus - Jiyuan-84       ............   ....LWS
AID16716.1 Bat SARS-like - Longquan-140      ............   ....LRS
ARI44799.1 Bat coronavirus - Anlong-103      ............   ....LRS
ARI44804.1 Bat coronavirus - Anlong-112      ............   ....LRS
AVP78042.1 bat-SL-CoVZXC21                   ............   ....LRS
AGC74176.1 Bat coronavirus Cp/Yunnan2011     ............   ....LRN
```

Figure 1.1   Alignments of coronavirus spike protein inserts. Amino acids are given in their one-letter form. The six inserts apart from the furin cleavage site (insert 6) are found in Zhou *et al.*, Extended Data Figure 3 (Amino acid sequence alignment of the S1 protein of the 2019-nCoV to SARS-CoV and selected bat SARS-CoVs) [13]. It should be noted that the sequence alignment was terminated just in front of the furin cleavage site. The contributions to additional high positive charge are found in four of the six inserts (red arrows) of the spike protein, and makes SARS-CoV-2 unique compared to other SARS-like coronaviruses found in nature.

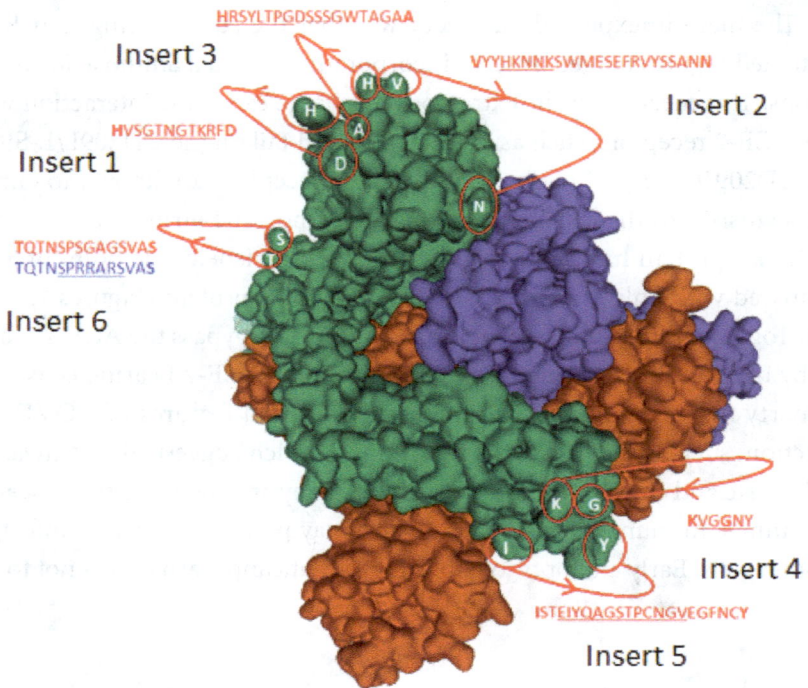

Figure 1.2   The identified inserts examined in the PDB 6VXX electron microscopy structure [34]. The sequences highlighted in red could not be found in the cryo-electron microscopy structure data. The six aligned sequences in Figure 1.1 are underlined in the missing sequences. Bold amino acids indicate first and last amino acids used to build the structure where the missing part is in between. Insert 6, the furin cleavage site, did not have the same sequence in 6VXX as in the reference Sars-CoV-2 sequence. The authors of the PDB 6VXX structure stated that a designed mutated strain lacking the furin cleavage site residues was used.

whole spike protein met with immediate rejection and the reason 'not in the public interest' from many journals, including *Nature*, *Science*, *The Lancet*, *Journal of Virology*, among others.

It was eventually published as part of an optimal design for a COVID-19 vaccine paper in *QRB Discovery* in June 2020. It has subsequently been downloaded more than 255,000 times [21].

We have subsequently investigated the history of GOF research, which could explain the more detailed origins of the SARS-CoV-2 virus (see Table 1.1).

Table 1.1   Gain of function history at the Wuhan Institute of Virology.

1	In 2010 scientists from the 'Special Viruses' section of the Wuhan Institute of Virology were engaged in gain of function experiments, jointly with international collaborators, to increase the infectiousness of coronaviruses for humans. What they did was, to put it simply, play about with bat and human ACE-2 receptors in order to train some SARS-like coronaviruses to adapt so that they could infect human cells more efficaciously [24, 25].
2	In 2015 scientists from the same 'Special Viruses' section of the Wuhan Institute of Virology were still engaged in gain of function work with a team from the University of North Carolina Chapel Hill. Together, they manipulated bat viruses to create a chimera, that is, an artificial man-made virus, called SHC014-MA15 which binds to and can proliferate on human upper airway cells. The lead Wuhan scientist, who provided the coronavirus material, was Dr Shi Zhengli. Properties described here are, in fact, what today the entire world would instantly recognise as those of COVID-19. In fact, *in vivo* experiments at Chapel Hill replicated the chimeric virus in mouse lungs which showed significant pathogenesis — the opposite of what the team had expected — but resembling the present COVID-19 virus. We can see, therefore, that the 2015 experiments advanced the 2010 work by perfecting in animal trials a virus optimised to infect the human upper respiratory tract. The 2015 authors were well aware that the chimeric virus which they had created was very dangerous because they discussed this fact [26]. They also speculated that *"review panels may deem similar studies too risky to pursue as increased pathogenicity in mammalian models cannot be excluded."* It is certainly the case that these experiments created a chimeric virus with very high infectivity and potentially targeted at the human upper respiratory tract [27, 28].
3	In 2018 Zhou *et al.* investigated a coronavirus outbreak associated with a fatal Swine Acute Diarrhoea Syndrome (SADS) in Guangdong Province (an epidemic in pigs) [29]. In summary, what this paper showed us is that this coronavirus used none of the three receptors it was expected to latch onto, including the well-known ACE-2, and was clearly utilising different ways of entering cells. At that point the scientists decided to dig into pig cells to discover which receptors the SADS coronavirus was using. They demonstrated considerable skills in this "hunt" for receptors and in testing them against a dangerous coronavirus.

The work can be summarised as follows. Several groups have used a viral backbone to insert different sequences to the RBD. Viruses can then be passaged in different cell lines so they can be enhanced for infecting cell lines from different species. However, it is very difficult to get bat samples to infect cell lines. Nevertheless, having sequenced many bat coronavirus genomes with none of them able to infect any cells nor animals, Becker and colleagues created a consensus chimeric virus transferring the human SARS spike RBD to the consensus BAT-ScoV backbone [24]. This allowed the virus to infect cells expressing the ACE-2 receptor, the primary receptor for the SARS virus. They also noted it could adapt to infect human epithelial cell cultures and in short use ligands other than ACE-2 for cell entry. More 'fine tuning' of binding efficiency to ACE-2 receptors was made using HIV/BJ01-S pseudovirus to express different ACE-2 receptors on human cell lines. The repeated passaging in these lines exposed them to cell surface receptors other than ACE-2 [25].

Dr Shi was in a team that successfully demonstrated the capability to interchange RBDs between bat coronavirus and human SARS viruses. They identified a sequence which converted non-ACE-2 binding to human ACE-2 binding [23]. There was a considerable amount of work by her team in optimising such virus chimeras to infect human cells. The collaboration with Ralph Baric and his team at Chapel Hill in the US is particularly noteworthy as he is an expert at RNA manipulation without leaving a trace [25].

What the Gain of Function Research Achieved

The ACE-2 receptor is required for SARS viruses to infect human cells. In addition, the inserts described by Sørensen *et al.* have added an extra charge, unlike any other SARS virus to date, which can allow the virus to latch onto the cell surface in the absence of the ACE-2 receptor [21]. Therefore, ACE-2 receptors have been inserted into different cells using viral vectors, including HIV. Whereas ACE-2 receptors are present on many cells, including epithelial cells in the lung and small intestine, endothelial cells, and smooth muscle cells, it was discovered that SARS-CoV-2 could initiate infection without the ACE-2 receptor such as the antigen-presenting cell receptors CD209L/L-SIGN [30]. Using specific cell lines, such as the primate VERO cell line and the human HeLa cell line, the viruses can be passaged not only to optimally bind to the ACE-2 receptor but to other receptors, such as those mentioned above.

Lu *et al.* [31] published in *The Lancet* of January 29, 2020 a paper with the title "Genomic characterisation and epidemiology of 2019 novel coronavirus: implications for virus origins and receptor binding" [31]. Here they show that the sequences of the new coronavirus are significantly different from other SARS-like viruses published at that point in time. This is in line with our observations linked to the additional net positive charge on SARS-CoV-2 S1 compared to the net negative charge on SARS-CoV-1 (2003). The main contributions to this elevated positive charge are the new sequence inserts found on the spike. Four (1,2,3 and 6) of the six inserts are located outside the RBD and are highly positively charged with pI = 11.00, 10.00, 8.76 and 12.06 and are all surface exposed, which make them well positioned to interact with other receptors such as CD209L/L-SIGN; see Figures 1.1 and 1.2.

We postulate that the FCS, together with the other five inserts, gives SARS-CoV-2 its extraordinary ability to infect many cell types and, combined with the high human sequence similarities, explains the main clinical pathologies that are seen. These include erythrocyte and lymphocyte depletion, infection of the nervous system, and interference with taste and smell, using receptors that also adversely affect innate immune cell function [21, 32].

Conclusions

The real mystery behind the origin of the virus is not that China and the initial WHO team tried to cover up the outbreak and suppress data that would actually have been useful to enforce the containment of COVID. It is not even the fact that the virus was more likely to have escaped a laboratory which had been reporting on successful GOF experiments for nearly a decade, than one that came from a cave naturally, 1,800 km away. No, it has to be the acceptance by politicians worldwide and their scientific advisors that China was right in that it is another zoonotic-like SARS-CoV-1 and that any other explanation must be ignored.

The WHO inspection of the origin Wuhan Institute, that was eventually demanded, was led by Dr Daszak and was totally controlled by the Chinese with regard to who could be included on the visiting team and what evidence could be looked at. This led to the misleading conclusion that a lab leak is unlikely, although it cannot be totally excluded. It should be remembered that the Chinese had destroyed all the evidence that could have been helpful, and had denied access to the serum samples of the early victims.

Thus, the whole world colluded in what some have called the 'death of science'. Matt Ridley in his excellent book *Viral* was astonished to find that senior Fellows of the Royal Society whom he questioned had not looked at the raw data because they considered it an obvious zoonotic jump [2]. Ridley set out to *show* it was a zoonotic leap, but concludes that it was more likely to have been a lab leak. He considers that we will never be able to prove this, as the evidence has been destroyed. What is surprising is that the GOF experiments being performed in Wuhan were in collaboration with American scientists and that the work was funded indirectly by the EcoHealth Alliance from the NIAID, of which the Director was Anthony Fauci, the most vociferous opponent of a laboratory origin. Stephen Quay, in his excellent book-length article on Bayesian analysis of all the evidence, agrees that a laboratory leak is over 99% the most likely origin [9]. This concluded beyond reasonable doubt that SARS-CoV-2 is not a natural zoonosis and is instead laboratory derived. A 170-page review of all the primary evidence is available on Zenodo [34]. When we weigh the balance of evidence available, a purely natural origin seems extremely unlikely.

Acknowledgements

Birger Sørensen helped write the details on our work in *QRB Discovery* and Professor Paul Goddard contributed many of the non-technical aspects, which he covered when writing his book *Pandemic* [32].

References

[1] Wang, L-F, Shi, Z, Zhang, S, *et al.* (2006). Review of bats and SARS. *Emerging Infectious Diseases*, **12**(12), 1834–1840.

[2] Chan, A & Ridley, M (2021). Chapter 3: The Wuhan Whistleblowers. In *Viral: The Search for the Origin of Covid-19*. 4th Estate.

[3] Goddard, PR (2020). *PANDEMIC: Plagues, Pestilence and War: A Personalised History*. Clinical Press Ltd.

[4] Zhou, P, Yang, XL, Wang, XG, *et al.* (2020). A pneumonia outbreak associated with a new coronavirus of probable bat origin. *Nature*, **579**, 270–273.

[5] Ge, X, Wang, N, Zhang, W, *et al.* (2016). Coexistence of multiple coronaviruses in several bat colonies in an abandoned mineshaft. *Virology Sinica*, **31**(1), 31–40.

[6] Rahalkar, MC & Bahulikar, RA (2022). Mojiang mine, RaTG13, miners' disease and related samples remain essential clues in the origin SARS-CoV-2. *Current Science*, **122**(3), 247.

[7] Zhou, P, Yang, X, Wang, XG, *et al.* (2020). Addendum: A pneumonia outbreak associated with a new coronavirus of probable bat origin. *Nature*, **588**, E6.

[8] Chan, A & Ridley, M (2021). Chapter 1: The Copper Mine. In *Viral: The Search for the Origin of Covid-19*. 4th Estate.

[9] Quay, S (2021). A Covid Bayesian Analysis. In Barnard, P, Quay, S and Dalgleish A (Eds.), *The Origin of the Virus: The Hidden Truths Behind the Microbe that Killed Millions of People*. Clinical Press Ltd.

[10] Andersen, KG, Rambaut, A, Lipkin, WI, *et al.* (2020). The proximal origin of SARS-CoV-2. *Nature Medicine*, **26**, 450–452.

[11] Calisher, C (2020). Statement in support of the scientists, public health professionals, and medical professionals of China combatting COVID-19. *The Lancet*, **395**, 10226.

[12] Birchall, S (2007, August 7). Defra must give us more hard facts. *The Guardian*. https://www.theguardian.com/uk/2007/aug/07/ruralaffairs.footandmouth.

[13] Zhou, P, *et al.* (2020). A pneumonia outbreak associated with a new coronavirus of probable bat origin. *Nature*, **579**, 270–273.

[14] Li, W, Wicht, O, van Kuppeveld, FJ, *et al.* (2015). A single point mutation creating a furin cleavage site in the spike protein renders porcine epidemic diarrhea coronavirus trypsin independent for cell entry and fusion. *Journal of Virology*, **89**(15), 8077–8081.

[15] Yang, Y, Liu, C, Du, L, *et al.* (2015). Two mutations were critical for bat-to-human transmission of Middle East Respiratory Syndrome coronavirus. *Journal of Virology*, **89**(17), 9119–9123.

[16] Zhou, H, Chen, X, Hu, T, *et al.* (2020). A novel bat coronavirus closely related to SARS-CoV-2 contains natural insertions at the S1/S2 cleavage site of the spike protein. *Current Biology*, **30**(11), 2196–2203.e3.

[17] Ambati, BK, Varshney, A, Lundstrom, K, *et al.* (2022). MSH3 homology and potential recombination link to SARS-CoV-2 furin cleavage site. *Frontiers in Virology*, **2**, 834808.

[18] Pollard, RB, Rockstroh, JK, Pantaleo, G, *et al.* (2014). Safety and efficacy of the peptide-based therapeutic vaccine for HIV-1, Vacc-4x: a phase 2 randomised, double-blind, placebo-controlled trial. *Lancet Infectious Diseases*, **14**(4), 291–300.

[19] Tseng, CT, Sbrana, E, Iwata-Yoshikawa, N, *et al.* (2012). Immunization with SARS coronavirus vaccines leads to pulmonary immunopathology on challenge with the SARS virus. *PLoS One*, **7**(4), e35421.

[20] Song, Z, Xu, Y, Bao, L, *et al.* (2019). From SARS to MERS, thrusting coronaviruses into the spotlight. *Viruses*, **11**(1), 59.

[21] Sørensen, B, Susrud, A & Dalgleish, AG (2020). Biovacc-19: a candidate vaccine for Covid-19 (SARS-Coronavirus-2) developed from analysis of its general method of action for infectivity. *QRB Discovery*, **1**, e6.

[22] Hamming, I, Timens, W, Bulthuis, MLC, *et al.* (2004). Tissue distribution of ACE2 protein, the functional receptor for SARS coronavirus. A first step in understanding SARS pathogenesis. *Journal of Pathology*, **203**, 631–637.

[23] Hou, Y, Peng, C, Yu, M, *et al.* (2010). Angiotensin-converting enzyme 2 (ACE2) proteins of different bat species confer variable susceptibility to SARS-Coronavirus entry. *Archives of Virology*, **155**, 1563–1569.

[24] Becker, MB, Graham, RL, Donaldson, EF, *et al.* (2008). Synthetic recombinant bat SARS-like coronavirus is infectious in cultured cells and in mice. *Proceedings of the National Academy of Sciences*, **105**(50), 19944–19949.

[25] Graham, RL & Baric, RS (2010). Recombination, reservoirs, and the modular spike: mechanisms of coronavirus cross-species transmission. *Journal of Virology*, **84**(7), 3134–3146.

[26] Menachery, VD, Yount, B, Debbink, K, *et al.* (2015). A SARS-like cluster of circulating bat coronaviruses shows potential for human emergence. *Nature Medicine*, **21**, 1508–1513.

[27] Menachery, VD, Yount, B, Sims, AC, *et al.* (2016). SARS-like WIV1-CoV poised for human emergence. *Proceedings of the National Academy of Sciences*, **113**(11), 3048–3053.

[28] Ren, W, Qu, X, Li, W, *et al.* (2008). Difference in receptor usage between Severe Acute Respiratory Syndrome (SARS) coronavirus and SARS-like coronavirus of bat origin. *Journal of Virology*, **82**(4), 1899–1907.

[29] Zhou, P, Fan, H, Lan, T, *et al.* (2018). Fatal swine acute diarrhoea syndrome caused by an HKU2-related coronavirus of bat origin. *Nature*, **556**, 255–258.

[30] Amraei, R, Yin, W, Napoleon, MA, *et al.* (2021). CD209L/L-SIGN and CD209/DC-SIGN act as receptors for SARS-CoV-2. *ACS Central Science*, **7**(7), 1156–1165.

[31] Lu, R, Zhao, X, Li, J, *et al.* (2020). Genomic characterisation and epidemiology of 2019 novel coronavirus: implications for virus origins and receptor binding. *The Lancet*, **395**(10224), 565–574.

[32] Workman, AD, Palmer, JN, Adappa, ND, *et al.* (2015). The role of bitter and sweet taste receptors in upper airway immunity. *Current Allergy and Asthma Reports*, **15**(12), 72.

[33] Quay, S (2021). A Bayesian analysis concludes beyond a reasonable doubt that SARS-CoV-2 is not a natural zoonosis but instead is laboratory derived. *Zenodo.* https://doi.org/10.5281/zenodo.4477081.

[34] Walls, AC, Park, Y-J, Tortorici, MA, *et al.* (2020). Structure, function, and antigenicity of the SARS-Coronavirus-2 spike glycoprotein. *Cell*, **181**(2), 281–292.e6.

Chapter

2

ChAdOx1: How an Academic Vaccine Achieved Global Reach

By Sean Elias

Summary

Developing, testing and licensing a vaccine in less than a year is an incredible achievement, but to do this as an academic institution adds to this triumph. In this chapter we start by discussing the work that helped lay the foundations for this success, notably the development of an accessible platform technology and the clinical infrastructure in place at the University of Oxford. We then move on to discuss how as academics we had to step out of our comfort zone and innovate, to ensure that our promising vaccine could join the global stage in the fight against the COVID-19 pandemic.

Introduction

My personal link to this story starts back in September 2008. I had just joined the Jenner Institute, a fresh Oxford undergraduate starting his first job. I was to be one of five founding members of the Institute's newest group, the 'Viral Vector Core Facility' (VVCF). The group was to be tasked with making pre-clinical adenoviral and Modified Vaccinia Ankara (MVA) viral vectored vaccines for the rest of the Institute, and with time for external orders as well. These vaccine platform technologies, standardised frameworks upon which novel vaccines could be developed, already sped up development, but were limited by the time which it took to train individuals to learn the techniques. The idea was that a core group and a manufacturing pipeline would further accelerate and improve the research pipeline. Students and Principal Investigators would no longer have to spend half their project making a single vaccine to test and the pipeline production system would allow several vaccines to be made at once to the same consistent specifications and standards. This would also aid to transition successful pre-clinical candidates to Good Manufacturing Practice (GMP) standard, with the VVCF linking up with the Clinical Biomanufacturing Facility (CBF), the University's GMP clinical grade manufacturing facility just down the road. As it turns out, both facilities would go on to play important roles just over 11 years later in 2020 at the start of the COVID-19 pandemic. On that first day, full of enthusiasm, I would never have predicted the journey that lay ahead of me or the amazing people I would meet and work with for years to come. One of those influential people I met that first day. Coming to the end of my introductory lab tour, I was introduced to a PhD student, who was also working on adenoviral vectors at the time. As the student stood up from the fridge full of plasmid constructs he promptly tipped the fullest tray all over the floor and under every fridge in the spill radius. Naturally I offered to help and we bonded over common interests. We have been friends ever since and I was best man at his wedding years later. This student, Matthew Dicks, went on to develop the ChAdOx1 viral vector used as the backbone for the Oxford/AstraZeneca COVID-19 vaccine [1].

Importance of Platform Technology

I think most vaccinologists would agree that the COVID-19 pandemic was the first proper opportunity for decades of research into vaccine platform technology to take centre stage. Before then mRNA vaccines were largely in pre-clinical development and most viral vectored vaccines were still only in early-stage human clinical trials. When the chips were down, these technologies made the first strong play and came up trumps. It is important to note that these newer technologies could well have failed at the first hurdle, and this could have set the platforms back a number of years. Instead, public interest and global investment in them would end up creating a watershed moment for future pandemic preparedness. Now, this is not to say all vaccines will and should be made this way in future. Platform technologies have their limitations, but their potential for flexibility, speed of development, transferability and low costs make them an attractive tool for researchers, especially those working on outbreak pathogens [2].

The adenoviral vectored vaccine platform has been the platform technology of choice at the Jenner Institute since its foundation. Adenoviruses, DNA-based viruses, were first used medically as recombinant vectors for gene therapy [3]. However, early studies suggested they may have characteristics more suited to use as vaccine vectors [4]. Adenoviruses have relatively large but easy-to-manipulate genomes and are easily rendered non-replicating for safety purposes by removal of the E1 region, whilst removal of an additional E3 region generates increased vector capacity for vaccine inserts up to 8 kb [5]. This is sufficient for most single vaccine transgene constructs but can also support smaller bivalent constructs as well.

With the removal of the E1 region, adenoviruses require complementary cell lines expressing the E1 gene for growth. The most common of these is the HEK293 cell line. Such cell lines are easy to handle, easily accessible and can be grown under static or suspension conditions, ideal for small- and large-scale production [6]. Genetic stability is also good over successive passages [7], essential for a commercial medicinal product.

Transgene expression, under the control of heterologous promotors, kickstarts the process of transcription and translation within host cells that results in vaccine antigen synthesis. During manufacture, this can be supressed using methods such as *tet* repression in specialist cell lines such as the HEK293-TRex line [8]. This has the benefit of increasing adenovirus yield, particularly in cases where the transgene product inhibits cellular growth. In human cells following vaccination, transgene expression is maintained alongside minimal viral gene expression [9].

Adenoviral vectors consistently induce both T-cell and antibody responses, and successive generations of adenoviral vectors have progressively driven stronger responses. Adenoviral vectors alone do not typically drive as strong an antibody response as some other genetic platform technologies despite utilising similar cellular mechanisms to generate immunity. Exactly why this is the case is the subject of recently initiated studies. Whilst single-dose adenovirus regimens have been shown to be effective, these vectors have consistently been shown to be more effective in prime boost regimens, either homologous or preferentially heterologous with a second adenovirus serotype or alternative viral vector such as MVA [2, 10].

There are thousands of potential adenoviruses that can be used as vectors and many of the first vectors were common human serotypes with broad tropism. Among these there are many different reasons as to why the potency of the vectored immune response may vary from vector to vector [11]. AdHu5 vectors, for example, are among the most potent, but their popularity dipped after the negative publicity from the STEP HIV trials [12]. Safety with human adenoviruses has otherwise been very good; however, human adenoviruses have one potential disadvantage: anti-vector immunity [13]. Human adenoviruses are one cause of common colds so we encounter them on a regular basis. In theory, an individual with pre-existing immunity against closely related adenoviruses to the vector of choice could have reduced vaccine-specific responses. In practice, evidence suggests that the effect is minor even with high anti-vector immunity from repeated natural exposure or vaccination.

To combat these theoretical concerns there was a systematic move in the field towards using non-human adenoviruses for which anti-vector immunity through exposure or cross-reactivity is negligible [14]. Chimpanzee adenoviruses have been the vectors of choice in this regard, as they are still effective at infecting humans [15]. Though chimpanzee vectors may have slightly reduced immunogenicity compared to the best human vectors, they have been shown to be effective at inducing comparable protection against disease in head-to-head studies [1].

One little discussed topic in regard to adenoviral vectors is patent ownership. Most vectors are owned by the company or institution that originally isolated and adapted the serovar as a vector. Whilst collaboration is common to allow different vectors to be used for different studies, legal agreements can slow down and limit progress if you are using someone else's vector. It was for this reason that the Jenner Institute and University of Oxford sought to develop our own viral vector platform over which we had complete control. This was a critical decision that would allow us to make our COVID-19 adenovirus-based vaccine globally accessible in the future.

The virus, now known as ChAdOx1, was first identified at Johns Hopkins University of Medicine and characterised in a publication from 1969 [16]. Originally called Y25, the virus was one of several adenoviruses isolated from the faeces of young chimpanzees who were being screened for hepatitis viruses. The University of Oxford used the sequence from the Y25 isolate in the development of the ChAdOx1 viral vector, with the process described in the following publication from 2012 [1].

Since then, ChAdOx1 has been used for the majority of new viral vectored vaccines at the Jenner Institute, particularly those for emerging and outbreak pathogens but also for some of our longer running programs such as malaria and tuberculosis. Several of these have progressed to phase I clinical trials, providing important safety and immunological data for the vector, justifying its continued status as our leading vaccine platform. A full list of our ChAdOx1 vaccines can be found in Table 2.1. Several of these have also shown the diverse utility of ChAdOx1. This includes a 'One Health' dual human/veterinary vaccine for Rift Valley Fever Virus [17], intranasal delivery as a tuberculosis vaccine [18] and capacity for holding stable bivalent constructs for Ebola.

Of these it was the ChAdOx1 vaccine program against MERS coronavirus which turned out to be highly valuable when it came to developing our COVID-19 vaccine. Firstly, we knew the spike protein of the MERS coronavirus was stable and effective in our ChAdOx1 viral vector [19, 20], and we predicted this was likely to translate to SARS-CoV-2 as well [21]. Secondly,

Table 2.1 ChAdOx1-based vaccine candidates developed by the Jenner Institute.

Pathogen	ChAdOx1 Vaccine Candidate	Stage of Development (CT: clinical trial)
MERS	ChAdOx1 MERS	Phase I/II CT
Lassa Virus	ChAdOx1 LASV	Pre-clinical
Nipah Virus	ChAdOx1 NiV	Pre-clinical
Rift Valley Fever Virus	ChAdOx1 RVF	Advanced veterinary, phase I human CT
Crimean Congo Haemorrhagic Fever Virus	Various	Pre-clinical
Ebola Virus	ChAdOx1 biEBOV	Phase I CT
Zika Virus	ChAdOx1 Zika	Phase I CT
Malaria	ChAdOx1 LS2	Phase I CT
Tuberculosis	ChAdOx1 85A	Phase I CT
Rabies	ChAdOx1 RabG	Phase I CT
Chikungunya	ChAdOx1 sCHIKV	Phase I CT
Plague	ChAdOx1 Plague	Phase I CT

from data from the MERS phase I human clinical trials [22] we knew that the type of immunogenicity induced (Th1) was likely to be effective and would not provoke antibody-dependant enhancement of disease, which was a concern during early research [23]. This meant that once the SARS-CoV-2 virus sequence was received in Jan 2020 and starter material developed, we could set up two parallel pathways, using VVCF to manufacture virus for the preclinical pipeline and the CBF for the clinical pipeline.

Importance of Clinical Trial Infrastructure

As an academic institution, the Jenner Institute has been well placed to research vaccines for historically difficult diseases (*e.g.*, malaria), or vaccines with little commercial interest such as neglected or rare diseases that only affect low- and middle-income countries (LMICs) and have limited geographical range (*e.g.*, Nipah virus, Lassa virus). With on-site manufacturing for pre-clinical and small batch clinical grade vaccines, we are well placed for running pre-clinical studies and small phase I and II clinical trials here in Oxford. However, Oxford is still a small city, even with a large population of students to target for clinical trials. A small trial of 100 volunteers could easily take months to recruit so over time we expanded to sites in Southampton and London to aid recruitment. As most of our vaccines were for tropical diseases, success meant running later-stage trials in endemic countries; so we have gradually built up a network of collaborating sites, for example in East and West Africa for malaria [24, 25] and South Africa for tuberculosis [26].

A watershed moment that changed the way we approached clinical trials in Oxford was the 2014/15 Ebola outbreak. Vaccines for Ebola did exist in 2014, but globally only four had completed phase I clinical trials and many were still in pre-clinical development [27]. A lack of funding and urgency had prevented them from being taken further down the clinical pipeline. However, because of Ebola's status as a potential target for bioterrorism, provision had been made by a few wealthy countries to hold stocks of these unlicensed vaccines to GMP standard, ready for use in humans. This meant that when the WHO made the call in 2014, clinical trials could start up rapidly using these stocks. The Jenner Institute in partnership with the Oxford Vaccine Group had the capacity in place to run clinical trials for a selection of these existing Ebola vaccines, which happened to be familiar viral vectors [28], despite not having developed our own. The first vaccine was given to volunteers just a month after the WHO's call. As it happens, I was a volunteer in this clinical trial and one of the first to receive a vaccine. One of the novelties of these studies was the way researchers and regulators worked together to shorten downtime and push through the vaccines to emergency approval as quickly as possible. This experience was undoubtedly of benefit for the time when this approach would be utilised again in the COVID-19 pandemic.

A major difference between the Ebola and COVID-19 pandemics was the fact that COVID-19 was global, and more importantly affected the world's economic powerhouses (US, EU, China, Russia). This single fact meant that global investment in development of COVID-19 vaccines was staggering. It also reveals the sad reality that diseases that only affect LMICs just are not taken as seriously by governments or pharmaceutical companies.

Despite this, it took a lot of campaigning to get finance secured for the development and testing of the Oxford vaccine. Initially the University put up capital, supplemented by small grants, for the work, but it was the UK Government who eventually provided the money to allow the work to continue [29]. This money also kickstarted progress on scaling up manufacture of the vaccine, something we will cover in detail later.

Money was not the only new challenge faced by the team during the pandemic. Previously, we were used to hosting up to 15 volunteers a day in clinic, limited by access to only a handful of clinic rooms. At the peak of the COVID-19 clinical trials we were hosting 120 volunteers. To allow such capacity we built temporary mobile clinics and drafted in additional nurses and doctors for vaccinations and follow-up appointments. In the lab one or two researchers working on a single clinical trial project might handle 10 clinical samples a day on a busy day and see them through from start to finish. With 120 samples you needed a team of 20 or more split into shifts and running as a production line to maximise efficiency. Even then you had people working to the early hours of the morning during the first few months. On top of this, we had to ensure everyone was fed and most importantly avoided catching and spreading the virus among the team. Thankfully, charitable donations meant we had food provided for us and miraculously, at the Jenner Institute at least, we avoided any outbreaks in the first phase of the pandemic — this was a real threat that could have undermined the project. Other challenges not previously faced included acquisition of basic items such as gloves, as we were competing with hospitals for personal protective equipment (PPE) at this point. On the IT front cybersecurity became a source of real concern as apparently nefarious forces wanted to steal our trial data. On top of this was the challenge of dealing with the media — something we as academics had little previous experience of.

For academics, presenting your work to the global media is not something you really expect to do unless you happen to have won a Nobel prize. Even a cutting-edge *Nature* or *Science* paper can be a difficult sell to the national press. During the pandemic this notion was turned on its head. Everyone wanted updates on our work on a daily basis. Unfortunately, this is not particularly compatible with clinical trials, where data collection takes time. Even just explaining the basic science behind the work was a challenge. I was amazed at how little basic understanding of vaccines there was initially among science journalists and editors, but to be fair, once they realised we were happy to help them if they asked (a concept I believe was new to them), we struck up some very positive relationships. Academia does afford you some freedom in this regard, but even so we had to carefully manage our messaging. At the start of the pandemic this was a challenge internally as our department did not really have the communications infrastructure to support the scale of the situation we were in. Only when the University's public affairs directorate stepped in and we developed an integrated support team of scientists, comms experts, content creators and social media managers did we truly get on top of the media situation. I personally believe the public appreciated the open and honest approach provided by scientists, particularly from our team and scientific advisors to the government, such as Chris Whitty and Jonathan Van-Tam. That is not to say it was plain sailing. Science and politics do not always mix and there were controversies and criticisms both avoidable and unavoidable, fair and unfair, throughout the pandemic. Either way, we are certainly more prepared to deal with this in the future.

Importance of Scaling up Manufacturing

The CBF at the University of Oxford has been providing GMP standard adenoviral vaccines for early-phase clinical trials for as long as the Jenner Institute has been working on them. A typical manufacturing batch could create between 100–1,000 doses, perfect for the typical phase I and II clinical trials run by the Jenner Institute. These batches were made using tried and tested traditional manufacturing methods including suspension cell shaker flasks and caesium chloride gradient ultracentrifugation [30]. It had been acknowledged that such methods were not really scalable; however, there was neither a pressing need or funding to incentivise development of alternatives. Most of the research and development at the CBF had instead focused on reducing the lead time from vaccine concept to vaccine seed stock for initial manufacturing [31].

The initial drive to make changes to adenovirus manufacturing at the Institute actually came from work into the development of a new rabies vaccine led by Dr Sandy Douglas and his group. Rabies is a disease that primarily affects LMICs nowadays but the only vaccines available are incredibly expensive, require multiple doses and are not widely accessible, meaning people often have to travel far to get access to them. Vaccines can cost the equivalent of a month's wages for some, so following a bite from a potentially rabid animal, such people are faced with an impossible decision — seek out a potentially lifesaving post-exposure vaccine or feed their family. With death from infection essentially guaranteed it is a dangerous gamble, and one that we estimate tens of thousands of people lose each year. If a new vaccine could be made that was cheaper and more widely accessible through scaled-up manufacture, fewer people would need to gamble with their lives. An adenovirus-based rabies vaccine could achieve this with some tweaking to the manufacturing process. As we were working with a platform technology any change driven by work on one disease could be directly applied to another, and as it turned out we had a pressing need to bring these changes through for our COVID-19 vaccine program.

The initial manufacturing changes were to move from 10 L shaker flasks to self-contained bioreactors and to replace ultracentrifugation with chromatography for purification. This significantly increased the yields of adenovirus obtained from the same size prep using traditional methods. Just as this work was being published [32], the COVID pandemic hit. As the reality sunk in that there was potentially a need for millions if not billions of doses, it was realised that we would need to go further with these changes. With a small, committed team working long hours this team managed not only to further improve yield but to ensure this increase was retained as the manufacturing was scaled up. We also had to look externally for help as we knew the CBF alone could not make enough vaccine, even with these changes, given the predicted demand.

Finding willing and able manufacturing partners with free capacity was no easy feat. You also have to remember that this was being done during a pandemic lockdown initially and that we were asking companies to collaborate on a project that was not going to generate huge profits. Those that signed on such as AstraZeneca are in my opinion not given enough credit for their decision to buy into our vision. The relationships forged and the lessons learnt from tech transfer are a big positive to come out of this pandemic. Less than two years after starting this process we now believe the method is refined enough to manufacture significant doses to respond to future pandemics in just 100 days [33]. But remember it is not just about how many doses we can make and how quickly we can make them, it is also about cost. In that regard it was the recruitment of the Serum Institute of India that had the biggest impact for making a vaccine for the world along the lines of the initial vision we had for rabies pre-pandemic.

A Look to the Future

There are some overarching questions to address here. Are we in a better position to address pandemics in the future? Are platform technologies the future of vaccine development? Is the academic vaccine model one that should be emulated? Can vaccine equity ever be truly achieved?

Following the 2014/15 Ebola pandemic there was an increased push to prepare for disease X. Whilst various initiatives stimulated progress towards pandemic preparedness, we were not truly prepared for when SARS-CoV-2 went global. If I am honest, scientists were probably expecting a smaller out-break of a deadlier but less globally transmissible virus, whilst governments were only really planning for the next influenza pandemic. We had the tech-nologies to quickly make vaccines, yes, but not really to scale up manufacture or distribute them. Now I believe scientists know where they went wrong but they still need the money to push this forward. We need to continue to identify new threats and have GMP seed stocks of new vaccines available. If possible, we need to have phase I clinical trials under our belts for these vac-cines. Though such trials are costly, they are significantly less so than phase II and III trials. Whilst governments made some verbal commitments to back such programs, I fear they may default on these as new global challenges arise. With the war in Ukraine and cost of living crisis, global spending priorities have already changed, even though the COVID-19 pandemic is not yet over and is still claiming lives in parallel.

One of the biggest lessons learnt from the pandemic is that more investment is needed in vaccine manufacturing. Whilst platform technologies allowed for rapid development of vaccines, little thought had been given on how to scale up manufacturing globally. Relying on manufacture in one country or by one company is clearly not sufficient and led to increasing political issues of vaccine nationalism and diplomacy. A solution to this is to build capacity for vaccine manufacture globally: first continentally then regionally and eventually to have a situation where countries can supply vaccines for their own populations. However, such a model requires a large initial investment and ongoing agreements for sharing of intellectual property and a non-profit or minimal profit approach when the stakes are high. Clearly these fit with an academic programme where vaccines are developed with public money, but are unlikely to be popular with pharmaceutical companies who need to make a profit to recover their initial investments — people often fail to understand how significant these can be. A single drug or vaccine can cost a company billions of pounds/dollars in research and development.

I believe a hybrid model where academics and pharmaceutical companies work together to develop vaccines is likely to become more commonplace in the future. It is not just a marriage of convenience; in the long run it benefits both parties and the public. This model allows academics to still have freedom to explore blue sky ideas but ultimately ensures that if an idea works, there is a natural pipeline to take it forward. For the companies, initial investments in or collaboration with academic institutions are relatively low cost, but can alleviate the financial risk when chasing high-risk research topics. Companies step back in once a vaccine looks promising, with the trade-off that as public funds were used for early research, they have to accept lower profits later on. This should in turn incentivise governments to invest in early vaccine research as expensive late-stage clinical trials costs are absorbed by companies and there is a promise of lower downstream buyer costs. Such collaborations also help encourage tech and staff transfer both ways between the public and private sectors. It is not a perfect model and the biggest challenge in my opinion is ensuring that such collaborations extend beyond the big players, be they companies, rich countries or universities, to ensure that stakeholders from LMICs are actively included.

Finally, what is the future of the ChAdOx1 vector? The ChAdOx1 COVID-19 vaccine will continue to play an important role in LMICs despite falling out of favour in Europe. The blood clot risk cited by many for this loss of favour has not carried the same weight in the rest of the world, thankfully. Despite the positives of mRNA vaccine technology, for some around the world this is still new and 'scary' tech and we must remember it equally has its own minor safety considerations, manifested as cases of myocarditis in young males. There is also seemingly more trust for something developed by a university over 'Big Pharma' in some parts of the world. Finally, cost will always be a major factor for poorer countries and the low cost of ChAdOx1 alongside our promise to keep it at cost in LMICs (whilst allowing for profit to be made from countries that can afford higher prices) will ensure it has a bright, short-term future. I say short term because I believe our vaccine will phase out of use for COVID. In time equally, low-cost vaccines such as more socially acceptable protein-in-adjuvant vaccines will become available and the cost for RNA vaccines will drop. There is also immunological justification for mixing and matching vaccine coverage to better boost immunity over reliance on just one vaccine.

I do not see this as a bad thing. ChAdOx1, and newer versions including ChAdOx2 [34], will continue to be perfect for new pandemic vaccines as well as for replacing older expensive vaccines such as for rabies, as highlighted above. Future versions will also benefit from further parallel technological advancements. One good example of this are studies into vector thermostability [35]. Studies have also shown that by freeze-drying adenovirus vectors onto sugar matrixes, there is potential for long-term stability at room temperature [36]. Another example is alternative delivery routes to needles to offer hope to those with trypanophobia (a surprisingly common reason for vaccine hesitancy). We have already tested our viral vector vaccines in aerosols [37] and nasal sprays [38] and even on microneedle patches [39] with some promise, though there is a long way to go before they are commonplace. These technologies may particularly benefit roll-out of vaccines in LMICs as they do not require the same level of training to deliver as traditional needle-based vaccines.

In conclusion, the future of vaccine development in academia and particularly Oxford is very promising. That said, we cannot rest on our laurels and must continue to chase funding to sustain many of the existing programs and push for new ones. With new global interest in our work, we can use this to our advantage to expand and we have done that. Already funding is coming in for new institutes and buildings in the form of the Pandemic Sciences Institute (PSI) and Poonwalla Vaccine Research Building. The vision of the PSI, where I now reside, very much fits the vision I describe above. It plans to bring together partners from academia, industry and public health organisations from across the world. It plans to create science-led innovations to accelerate the understanding and to develop new diagnostics, treatments, vaccines and digital disease control tools. And finally, it plans to achieve this with a focus on equitable access of benefits for all. I look forward to being a part of this vision.

Acknowledgements

Firstly I would like to thank Professor Dame Sarah Gilbert for her support both in shaping my current role within the Institute and for her ongoing acknowledgement of the importance of public engagement and science communication. I would also like to thank Sue Morris and Amjad Parkar for reviewing the content of this chapter and editorial input, and Adam Ritchie for providing information for the section on manufacturing. Finally I would like to thank my friend Matthew Dicks for making ChAdOx1 in the first place.

References

[1] Dicks, MD, *et al.* (2012). A novel chimpanzee adenovirus vector with low human sero-prevalence: improved systems for vector derivation and comparative immunogenicity. *PLoS One*, **7**(7), e40385.

[2] Ewer, K, *et al.* (2017). Chimpanzee adenoviral vectors as vaccines for outbreak pathogens. *Human Vaccines and Immunotherapeutics*, **13**(12), 3020–3032.

[3] Wilson, JM (1996). Adenoviruses as gene-delivery vehicles. *New England Journal of Medicine*, **334**(18), 1185–1187.

[4] Tatsis, N & Ertl, HC (2004). Adenoviruses as vaccine vectors. *Molecular Therapy*, **10**(4), 616–629.

[5] Mizuguchi, H, Kay, MA & Hayakawa, T (2001). Approaches for generating recombinant adenovirus vectors. *Advanced Drug Delivery Reviews*, **52**(3), 165–176.

[6]   Morris, SJ, *et al.* (2016). Laboratory-scale production of replication-deficient adenovirus vectored vaccines. *Methods in Molecular Biology*, **1349**, 121–135.

[7]   Cottingham, MG, *et al.* (2012). Preventing spontaneous genetic rearrangements in the transgene cassettes of adenovirus vectors. *Biotechnology and Bioengineering*, **109**(3), 719–728.

[8]   Gall, JG, *et al.* (2007). Rescue and production of vaccine and therapeutic adenovirus vectors expressing inhibitory transgenes. *Molecular Biotechnology*, **35**(3), 263–273.

[9]   Almuqrin, A, *et al.* (2021). SARS-CoV-2 vaccine ChAdOx1 nCoV-19 infection of human cell lines reveals low levels of viral backbone gene transcription alongside very high levels of SARS-CoV-2 S glycoprotein gene transcription. *Genome Medicine*, **13**(1), 43.

[10] Draper, SJ & Heeney, JL (2010). Viruses as vaccine vectors for infectious diseases and cancer. *Nature Reviews in Microbiology*, **8**(1), 62–73.

[11] Coughlan, L (2020). Factors which contribute to the immunogenicity of non-replicating adenoviral vectored vaccines. *Frontiers in Immunology*, **11**, 909.

[12] Fitzgerald, DW, *et al.* (2011). An Ad5-vectored HIV-1 vaccine elicits cell-mediated immunity but does not affect disease progression in HIV-1-infected male subjects: results from a randomized placebo-controlled trial (the Step study). *Journal of Infectious Diseases*, **203**(6), 765–772.

[13] Mennechet, FJD, *et al.* (2019). A review of 65 years of human adenovirus seroprevalence. *Expert Reviews in Vaccines*, **18**(6), 597–613.

[14] Nebie, I, *et al.* (2014). Assessment of chimpanzee adenovirus serotype 63 neutralizing antibodies prior to evaluation of a candidate malaria vaccine regimen based on viral vectors. *Clinical and Vaccine Immunology*, **21**(6), 901–903.

[15] Morris, SJ, *et al.* (2016). Simian adenoviruses as vaccine vectors. *Future Virology*, **11**(9), 649–659.

[16] Hillis, WD & Goodman, R (1969). Serologic classification of chimpanzee adenoviruses by hemagglutination and hemagglutination inhibition. *Journal of Immunology*, **103**(5), 1089–1095.

[17] Stedman, A, *et al.* (2019). Safety and efficacy of ChAdOx1 RVF vaccine against Rift Valley fever in pregnant sheep and goats. *NPJ Vaccines*, **4**, 44.

[18] Pinpathomrat, N, *et al.* (2021). Using an effective TB vaccination regimen to identify immune responses associated with protection in the murine model. *Vaccine*, **39**(9), 1452–1462.

[19] Alharbi, NK, *et al.* (2017). ChAdOx1 and MVA based vaccine candidates against MERS-CoV elicit neutralising antibodies and cellular immune responses in mice. *Vaccine*, **35**(30), 3780–3788.

[20] van Doremalen, N, *et al.* (2020). A single dose of ChAdOx1 MERS provides protective immunity in rhesus macaques. *Science Advances*, **6**(24), eaba8399.

[21] Watanabe, Y, *et al.* (2021). Native-like SARS-CoV-2 spike glycoprotein expressed by ChAdOx1 nCoV-19/AZD1222 vaccine. *ACS Central Science*, **7**(4), 594–602.

[22] Bosaeed, M, *et al.* (2022). Safety and immunogenicity of ChAdOx1 MERS vaccine candidate in healthy Middle Eastern adults (MERS002): an open-label, non-randomised, dose-escalation, phase 1b trial. *Lancet Microbe*, 3(1), e11-e20.

[23] Lee, WS, *et al.* (2020). Antibody-dependent enhancement and SARS-CoV-2 vaccines and therapies. *Nature Microbiology*, 5(10), 1185–1191.

[24] Datoo, MS, *et al.* (2021). Efficacy of a low-dose candidate malaria vaccine, R21 in adjuvant Matrix-M, with seasonal administration to children in Burkina Faso: a randomised controlled trial. *Lancet*, 397(10287), 1809–1818.

[25] Ogwang, C, *et al.* (2015). Prime-boost vaccination with chimpanzee adenovirus and modified vaccinia Ankara encoding TRAP provides partial protection against Plasmodium falciparum infection in Kenyan adults. *Science Translational Medicine*, 7(286), 286re5.

[26] Ndiaye, BP, *et al.* (2015). Safety, immunogenicity, and efficacy of the candidate tuberculosis vaccine MVA85A in healthy adults infected with HIV-1: a randomised, placebo-controlled, phase 2 trial. *Lancet Respiratory Medicine*, 3(3), 190–200.

[27] Marzi, A & Feldmann, H. (2014). Ebola virus vaccines: an overview of current approaches. *Expert Reviews in Vaccines*, 13(4), 521–531.

[28] Milligan, ID, *et al.* (2016). Safety and immunogenicity of novel adenovirus type 26- and Modified Vaccinia Ankara-vectored Ebola vaccines: a randomized clinical trial. *JAMA*, 315(15), 1610–1623.

[29] Cross, S, *et al.* (2021). Who funded the research behind the Oxford-AstraZeneca COVID-19 vaccine? *BMJ Global Health*, 6(12), e007321.

[30] Su, Q, Sena-Esteves, M & Gao, G (2019). Purification of the recombinant adenovirus by cesium chloride gradient centrifugation. *Cold Spring Harbor Protocols*, 2019(5), prot095547.

[31] Gilbert, S & Green, C (2021). *Vaxxers: A Pioneering Moment in Scientific History*. Hodder & Stoughton.

[32] Fedosyuk, S, *et al.* (2019). Simian adenovirus vector production for early-phase clinical trials: A simple method applicable to multiple serotypes and using entirely disposable product-contact components. *Vaccine*, 37(47), 6951–6961.

[33] Joe, CCD, *et al.* (2022). Manufacturing a chimpanzee adenovirus-vectored SARS-CoV-2 vaccine to meet global needs. *Biotechnology and Bioengineering*, 119(1), 48–58.

[34] Folegatti, PM, *et al.* (2019). Safety and immunogenicity of a novel recombinant simian adenovirus ChAdOx2 as a vectored vaccine. *Vaccines (Basel)*, 7(2), 40.

[35] Berg, A, *et al.* (2021). Stability of chimpanzee adenovirus vectored vaccines (ChAdOx1 and ChAdOx2) in liquid and lyophilised formulations. *Vaccines (Basel)*, 9(11), 1249.

[36] Dulal, P, *et al.* (2021). Characterisation of factors contributing to the performance of nonwoven fibrous matrices as substrates for adenovirus vectored vaccine stabilisation. *Scientific Reports*, 11(1), 20877.

[37] Riste, M, *et al.* (2021). Phase I trial evaluating the safety and immunogenicity of candidate TB vaccine MVA85A, delivered by aerosol to healthy M.tb-infected adults. *Vaccines (Basel)*, 9(4), 396.

[38] Green, CA, *et al.* (2019). Novel genetically-modified chimpanzee adenovirus and MVA-vectored respiratory syncytial virus vaccine safely boosts humoral and cellular immunity in healthy older adults. *Journal of Infection*, **78**(5), 382–392.

[39] Pearson, FE, *et al.* (2015). Induction of CD8(+) T cell responses and protective efficacy following microneedle-mediated delivery of a live adenovirus-vectored malaria vaccine. *Vaccine*, **33**(28), 3248–3255.

Chapter

3

mRNA Vaccines: From Lab Concept to Leading Rescue Platform During the COVID-19 Pandemic

By Hana Hassanin

Summary

This chapter sheds light on the milestones and history of mRNA vaccine development. The challenges encountered with an mRNA-based vaccine, and how MERS (Middle East Respiratory Syndrome) and SARS (Severe Acute Respiratory Syndrome) impacted the success of finding quick and effective vaccines, are described. I show how an already existing platform was modified to target the new coronavirus pathogen, and what factors played a crucial role in public acceptance or refusal of the RNA-based vaccines.

Introduction

History teaches us that great innovation and creative solutions come to light during a crisis. This has been experienced across various realms such as economy, industry, engineering, defence, transport, social sciences and many more. Medicine and healthcare are not an exception. In fact, there have been several lifesaving and breakthrough innovations that were materialised and introduced during a health crisis.

The American biochemist and pharmacologist, Getrude B Elion, once said: "I had fallen in love with a young man, and we were planning to get

35

married. And then he died of subacute bacterial endocarditis. Two years later with the advent of penicillin, he would have been saved. It reinforced in my mind the importance of scientific discovery" [1]. There is a wealth of medical discoveries in history that shaped today's life; from the unearthing of penicillin that saved thousands of soldiers' lives during World War II, to the eradication of polio infection by the invention of polio vaccines.

The pressure of finding, testing, and applying medical solutions that are effective in addressing a particular health problem can be hugely challenged by the nature of this health problem. Infectious diseases are one of the most challenging areas in this regard.

One of the obvious challenging characteristics of infectious diseases is the potential of an unpredictable global pandemic scenario. This is in addition to several other factors such as transmissibility, dependence on the nature of human behaviours, the need of preventing infection in close contacts and communities, pathogen evolution, diversity of human host immunity, and nature of disease acuteness with relatively quick outcome of dying or recovering spontaneously [2].

The acute and unpredictable nature of infectious diseases necessitates the continuous collaborative work of scientists, physicians, and the pharmaceutical industry to ensure preparedness for an endemic and pandemic calamity. This does not necessarily mean the presence of a pathogen-specific or target-specific solution; rather it means a well-researched platform that can be easily used and speedily tailored in an unexpected global pandemic.

As the whole world was confronted by the COVID-19 pandemic in 2020, it became crucial to excavate effective solutions very swiftly to gain control of the world's biggest crisis since World War II. Very soon, the glimmer of hope, in the journey of overcoming COVID-19 infection and its impact, became a life-changing reality as two mRNA COVID-19 vaccines were approved and ready to be widely administered.

This chapter will go through the milestones of mRNA vaccine[s] development, the challenges encountered using this mRNA-based vaccine concept, how MERS and SARS impacted the success of finding quick and effective vaccines, how an already existing platform was modified to target the new pathogen, and what factors played a crucial role in public acceptance or refusal of the RNA-based vaccines.

History of mRNA Vaccines

In January 2020, the WHO announced the COVID-19 outbreak as a Public Health Emergency of International Concern [3]. Soon after, in March 2020, COVID-19 was declared a global pandemic based on the WHO assessment [4].

Only after about eight months from the COVID-19 outbreak, two vaccines were authorised and ready to be administered to the population to prevent severe COVID-19 cases, decrease COVID-19-related hospitalisation, and minimise the spread of the infection.

The two vaccines, namely the Pfizer-BioNTech and the Moderna COVID-19 vaccines, were one of the very first potential candidates that entered clinical development during the COVID-19 pandemic. Both vaccines are mRNA-based vaccines and have demonstrated around 95% efficacy in their phase III clinical trials [5].

The world drama of combating the COVID-19 pandemic has not only changed every aspect of life but has raised many questions about what seemed to be the rescue solution in bringing it to an end. Questions, doubts, discussions, misconception and misinformation characterised the past two years since the beginning of the pandemic.

Is the mRNA-based concept a new technology that has only emerged due to the need during the COVID-19 pandemic? The answer is "No". There is a long history behind the discovery of mRNA-based technology, which started as early as the 1960s [6]. This was followed by dedicated research into developing the delivery method of mRNA into cells, which was commenced in the 1970s. Transfecting mRNA was one of the main stumbling blocks in applying this new technology due to the highly degradable nature of RNA and consequently its need for a suitable vehicle to get it transported intactly into the cells. This hurdle meant that the promising approach was not able to proceed further until the solution appeared with advances made in nanotechnology. The landmark experiment was performed by Robert Malone, a graduate student at the Salk Institute for Biological Studies in La Jolla, California, in late 1987. Malone used synthetic lipid particles that enveloped mRNA and enabled efficient and reproducible RNA transfection [7]. In his publication in 1989, Malone wrote: "the procedure can be used to efficiently transfect RNA into human, rat, mouse, *Xenopus*, and *Drosophila* cells" [7]. Malone believed that his successful experiment meant the potential of using RNA as a treatment for medical conditions. Malone described this in notes he wrote down on 11 January 1988 where he stated "it might be possible to treat RNA as a drug" [6]. The proof of concept of his approach was achieved later in the same year by another experiment that showed successful transfection of liposome-based mRNA into frog embryos; this was the first mRNA transfection in a living organism [6].

People may wonder why we have not heard much about mRNA-based vaccines prior to the COVID-19 pandemic. Were there any mRNA vaccines? In what therapeutic areas were mRNA-based molecules first tested? To answer these questions, it is essential to understand that a considerable amount of time was needed (1960s–1990) to develop the novel mRNA-based molecules into easily deliverable and suitably designed agents. It has been a continuous process of improvement and modification of mRNA agents to refine delivery in the cells, enhance stability and reduce immune response against them by the body immune system. The last two decades (1990–2019) marked the active phase of testing these molecules as therapeutic agents in variant areas such as genetic illnesses, cancers, and infectious diseases [8]. In 1990, a direct gene transfer into mouse muscle was the first proof of concept and can be considered as the foundation of mRNA-therapeutic principle [9]. The first mRNA vaccine, that encoded human carcinoembryonic antigen (CEA), was developed in 1995 to examine the feasibility of utilising a mRNA vector as a cancer vaccine. This founded the strategy of using mRNA vaccines as immunogenic agents against proto-oncogenes with the vision of decreasing the risk of malignancy induced by prolonged expressions of specific proteins [10]. This was followed by a flux of cancer immunotherapy pre-clinical and clinical trials conducted using mRNA vaccines in 1999, 2002, 2009 and 2010 [11–14]. At the same time, further mRNA vaccine clinical trials were applied to other therapeutic areas such as rabies in 2017 and HIV in 2018 and 2019 [15–17]. Moreover, mRNA vaccines were tested in pre-clinical and clinical trials for respiratory syncytial virus, herpes virus, dengue virus and lethal Nipah virus [18–21].

It was not down to luck nor coincidence that the first two authorised COVID-19 mRNA vaccines were invented and developed by BioNTech and Moderna companies. Tracing back the history of both companies sets a very clear picture that their mRNA vaccine is not a newborn; rather it is years of commitment, knowledge accumulation and trials performed on this very specific platform. Looking at the BioNTech history, as an example, shows that they started in 2007 engineering RNA to improve genetic vaccines and enhance the induction of immune response [22]. In 2012, BioNTech started their first early phase I clinical trial on RNA immunotherapy in melanoma: an approach known now as the FixVac approach. It was then followed by another phase I clinical trial with RNA individualised immunotherapy (iNeST) in 2013 [23]. They published their first results of an intravenously administered mRNA clinical trial in 2016 [24]. The latter was the start of a series of other published results of mRNA clinical trials in 2017 [25]. With this rich profile of mRNA-centred research, Pfizer-BioNTech started what is called "Project Lightspeed" to speedily develop a safe and effective vaccine that gave birth to the very first mRNA COVID-19 vaccine which received emergency use of authorisation following a worldwide phase III clinical trial [26]. Likewise, Moderna has an affluent history in pioneering and testing mRNA-based therapeutics [6]. Both Moderna and BioNTech have been seen as heroes of the COVID-19 pandemic. It is very disturbing to see that Moderna is filing patent infringement lawsuits against BioNTech and Pfizer claiming that they have used Moderna's pioneered mRNA platform technology [27]. Will this influence the BioNTech/Pfizer vaccine accessibility in the future? Will there be an impact on BioNTech/Pfizer's plan of refining their current vaccine to face new variants of the virus? How will the public see this conflict and what impact will it have on the companies' credibility? All these are pertinent questions that currently have no answers and only time will tell.

SARS and MERS Outbreaks

Undoubtedly, the speed of developing COVID-19 vaccines during the pandemic was remarkable. Although the availability of the mRNA-based platform was a main facilitator, there have been other crucial factors that constituted the groundwork of the vaccines' rapid development. One of the pivotal factors was understanding the structure and pathogenicity of the COVID-19 causative agent. SARS-CoV-2 (Severe Acute Respiratory Syndrome Coronavirus-2), the causative agent for COVID-19, is a member of the coronavirus bigger family. Members of the coronavirus family are related, share similar structure, and cause respiratory symptoms that range from mild to life-threatening in humans [28]. More knowledge about coronaviruses has been cultivated for almost two decades since the emergence of SARS in Southern China in 2002, and MERS in the Arabian Peninsula and in South Korea in 2012. MERS and SARS are caused by MERS-CoV and SARS-CoV, both of which possess similar structure and pathogenic profile with SARS-CoV-2. Several vaccine modalities were designed to target SARS-CoV and MERS-CoV. These vaccines were also tested in pre-clinical models but only a few made it to the clinical trial phase, and none gained FDA approval [28]. Whilst there was no success in progressing and approving a vaccine in the case of SARS and MERS, the already tested vaccine approaches underpinned the rapid development, testing, and approval of COVID-19 vaccines. The accessible knowledge of the spike protein (S-protein) and its importance in the virus's pathogenicity was a main stone in paving the way for the whole process. Considering the biological similarity, the COVID-19 vaccine development strategy has benefited enormously from the available results in using the S-protein in its full length or subunits in trialled vaccines to target SARS-CoV and MERS-CoV [28]. In Feb 2020, Chinese scientists sequenced the genome of the COVID-19 virus [29]. The clinical lesson learned from SARS-CoV and MERS-CoV, together with the well-researched mRNA platform and the known S-protein genome sequence, sculpted a golden triangle that guided the expeditious COVID-19 mRNA vaccine development programme. The scientific community, supported by phenomenal collaboration between academic institutions, governments, and the pharmaceutical industry, crowned their effort with unprecedented speed in an unprecedented pandemic.

A New Era in Vaccinology

Prior to the COVID-19 pandemic, in 2018, *Nature Reviews Drug Discovery* published a detailed review of mRNA vaccines, which discussed mRNA vaccines platform, its application, previous experience, challenges, future, and the consideration of a new era in vaccinology founded by these promising vaccines [30]. Now, after living through the COVID-19 pandemic, a requisite critical assessment of relevant aspects is needed. Was the pandemic a real-life test of the claimed benefits for the mRNA vaccine concept? Has the pandemic's challenging environment been the golden opportunity in progressing the mRNA vaccine concept to a lead position?

With the fast-evolving COVID-19 pandemic, high pathogenicity and transmissibility of the virus, terrifying numbers of hospitalisation, increasing figures of death and major socioeconomic upheaval, the global foremost priority was to secure an effective and safe vaccine at light speed.

The mRNA vaccine concept was an ideal first solution to be examined based on many favourable characteristics. In developing a vaccine quickly, a fast-track process is needed at multiple levels: designing, manufacturing, testing and lastly authorising the vaccine. The flexibility of the mRNA vaccine platform enabled a quick and easy molecular design by inserting the genomic sequence of the S-protein. There was no need to spend months in culturing the virus in mammalian cells, inactivating the virus, and then purifying the vaccine as is the case in many traditional vaccine approaches. Manufacturing of the designed vaccines proved to be easily applied on a large scale for clinical use [31]. The cost effectiveness is still unclear as the production relies on the use of expensive and limited materials [31].

In terms of safety, mRNA vaccines contain no killed or attenuated virus which may theoretically mean they are safer than other conventional vaccine approaches that contain virus or viral materials. In the era of precision medicine, the mRNA vaccine approach has another added value of precisely introducing a specific protein genomic sequence that is carefully selected based on the virus pathogenicity mechanism of action. The body cells act as a factory that translate this genomic sequence (mRNA) into multiple copies of the targeted protein (S-protein in the case of COVID-19 vaccines), which in turn trigger the body immune system to produce immunity against this specific target.

The prevalence of COVID-19 during the pandemic was an ideal milieu to conduct large-scale global clinical trials to test safety and efficacy. Within days from the identification of COVID-19 in Dec 2019, the SARS-CoV-2 genome was sequenced. After about two months, the mRNA COVID-19 vaccine candidates entered phase I clinical trial and a few months later phase III clinical trials were up and running. Both frontrunning mRNA vaccines, Pfizer-BioNTech and Moderna, demonstrated high and acceptable tolerance and safety profiles [32].

The highly flexible and adaptive mRNA-based concept has inspired another novel RNA-based vaccine called the saRNA vaccine (self-amplifying RNA vaccine). The saRNA has a self-replicant nature which leads to production of high copies of the antigen while using a low dose of the vaccine. saRNA vaccine is inherently self-adjuvating which can trigger broader immunogenicity with less added adjuvants and with lower dose [33]. A COVID-19 phase I First in Human study was commenced in 2020 using encapsulated saRNA COVID-19 candidate (LNP-nCoVsaRNA) developed by scientists in Imperial College London. The vaccine was found safe for clinical development and is immunogenic at low dose levels. Modifications of this novel vaccine have been deemed necessary to optimise humoral responses and reach its potential as an effective vaccine against SARS-CoV-2 [34]. Clinical trials are still ongoing.

The success of mRNA vaccines in COVID-19 is a testimonial of the effectiveness and the practicality of this technology. The COVID-19 pandemic was an accelerating factor to put this novel concept into action and verify it in applied medicine. This may give more assurance that the world will be better prepared for the next pandemic. Nevertheless, the journey has just started, and many questions need to be addressed to be better equipped for the future. We need clearer insight and answers to many questions: how to modify mRNA vaccines to target the ever-changing variants of the virus, ways to develop multivalent vaccines, how to tackle immune escape, determine the length of immunity, the ideal number of vaccinations and boosters needed per year to achieve good immunity, data about vaccine immunogenicity status in a non-pandemic environment and host-tolerance concern all ought to be looked at.

What Caused Public Hesitancy in Accepting mRNA Vaccines?

Myths, misinformation and even disinformation distinguished the COVID-19 pandemic period. One can blame social media where there are no rules, scrutiny, or control on the shared information and anyone can say anything. Of course, this has hugely contributed to shaping the public opinion about trusting vaccines that have been authorised in less than a year rather than the conventional 5–10-year period it usually takes.

The public has been kept in the dark all the years as the mRNA-based concept was under development. They were not aware of the bevy of accumulated knowledge and trials that assembled the ripe platform. The public hesitancy is justifiable by the lack of awareness of the history behind these novel discoveries. The public has not been enlightened of the phenomenal speed the regulatory authorities worked at to prioritise the COVID-19 vaccine development and approval process. There were no cut corners but rather a creative new approach to streamline, improve and adapt the whole process. In fact, the way and speed by which the vaccine development and approval have been conducted was one of the great life lessons on which authorities are now building to readjust and enhance clinical trials in an effective and less lengthy approach while preserving a high standard. Scientists and medical professionals have a responsibility to apprise the public about drug development processes and discoveries. There are so many lessons to be learnt from the pandemic, and keeping the public at the heart of science is one of the most important.

On a positive note, public involvement in clinical trials has been boosted by the pandemic. Clinical trials have always been the foremost way to validate new therapeutics. A promising vaccine will never find its way to prevent or treat diseases if not properly tested in strictly controlled clinical trials. The latter will never materialise without the willingness of the public and communities to help science and to participate in order to enable the collection of reliable data. Recruiting participants in early phases (First in Human and phase I) has never been an easy job. It is quite difficult to recruit participants for a trial to test a medication for a disease that is not relevant to them. The pandemic propelled the importance of clinical trials to the spotlight and made it relevant to almost everyone and acceptable by many in the public domain. People became more interested in learning about the virus, the vaccines and more willing to be part of the vaccine development process by getting enrolled in clinical trials. This interest and relevance augmented the recruitment process to clinical trials which added a faster step towards approving the vaccine. It gave a better opportunity to understand how important it is to be part of the scientific and medical community without the need to be a scientist or a physician.

Conclusion

When Victor Hugo defined history, he said: "What is history? An echo of the past in the future; a reflex from the future on the past". The history of scientific work on a mRNA-based approach has clearly echoed in the COVID-19 pandemic era. Without this history, we would have not been able to achieve what has been realised in a very short time. The mRNA concept has been proved successful and has passed the test in practical terms. We may end up with the biggest real-world data in history which will surely guide the path for further refinement to ensure higher efficacy and safety of vaccines. The future may still carry many surprises and more pandemics, but surely the world is better prepared. Observing the voyage of mRNA, from lab concept to leading rescue platform during the COVID-19 pandemic, is a boost of confidence to the scientific and medical community but also to the public as a whole.

References

[1] Núñez Valdés, J, de Pablos Pons, F & Ramos Carrillo, A (2022). Gertrude Belle Elion, chemist and pharmacologist, discoverer of highly relevant active substances. *Foundations*, **2**(2), 443–456.

[2] Fauci, AS & Morens, DM (2012). The perpetual challenge of infectious diseases. *New England Journal of Medicine*, **367**(1), 89–90.

[3] WHO Emergency Committee (2020, January 30). Statement on the second meeting of the International Health Regulations (2005) Emergency Committee regarding the outbreak of novel coronavirus (2019-nCoV). *WHO*. https://www.who.int/news/item/30-01-2020-statement-on-the-second-meeting-of-the-international-health-regulations-(2005)-emergency-committee-regarding-the-outbreak-of-novel-coronavirus-(2019-ncov).

[4] Ghebreyesus, TA (2020, March 11). WHO Director-General's opening remarks at the media briefing on COVID-19. *WHO*. https://www.who.int/director-general/speeches/detail/who-director-general-s-opening-remarks-at-the-media-briefing-on-covid-19---11-march-2020.

[5] Polack, FP, Thomas, SJ, Kitchin, N, *et al.* (2020). Safety and efficacy of the BNT162b2 mRNA Covid-19 vaccine. *New England Journal of Medicine*, **383**(27), 2603–2615.

[6] Dolgin, E (2021). The tangled history of mRNA vaccines. *Nature*, **597**(7876), 318–324.

[7] Malone, RW, Felgner, PL & Verma, IM (1989). Cationic liposome-mediated RNA transfection. *Proceedings of the National Academy of Sciences*, **86**(16), 6077–6081.

[8] Qin, S, Tang, X, Chen, Y, Chen, K, Fan, N, Xiao, W, Zheng, Q, Li, G, Teng, Y, Wu, M & Song, X (2022). mRNA-based therapeutics: powerful and versatile tools to combat diseases. *Signal Transduction and Targeted Therapy*, **7**(1), 166.

[9] Wolff, JA, Malone, RW, Williams, P, Chong, W, Acsadi, G, Jani, A & Felgner, PL (1990). Direct gene transfer into mouse muscle in vivo. *Science*, **247**(4949), 1465–1468.

[10] Conry, RM, Curiel, DT, Smith, B & LoBuglio, AF (1995). Immune response to intramuscular or intravenous CEA polynucleotide immunization in large animal models. *Journal of Immunotherapy*, **18**(2), 134.

[11] Zhou, WZ, Hoon, D, Huang, S, Fujii, S, Hashimoto, K, Morishita, R & Kaneda, Y (1999). RNA melanoma vaccine: induction of antitumor immunity by human glycoprotein 100 mRNA immunization. *Human Gene Therapy*, **10**(16), 2719–2724.

[12] Heiser, A, Coleman, D, Dannull, J, Yancey, D, Maurice, MA, Lallas, CD, Dahm, P, Niedzwiecki, D, Gilboa, E & Vieweg, J (2002). Autologous dendritic cells transfected with prostate-specific antigen RNA stimulate CTL responses against metastatic prostate tumors. *Journal of Clinical Investigation*, **109**(3), 409–417.

[13] Weide, B, Pascolo, S, Scheel, B, Derhovanessian, E, Pflugfelder, A, Eigentler, TK, Pawelec, G, Hoerr, I, Rammensee, HG & Garbe, C (2009). Direct injection of protamine-protected mRNA: results of a phase½2 vaccination trial in metastatic melanoma patients. *Journal of Immunotherapy*, **32**(5), 498–507.

[14] Kreiter, S, Selmi, A, Diken, M, Koslowski, M, Britten, CM, Huber, C, Türeci, Z & Sahin, U (2010). Intranodal vaccination with naked antigen-encoding RNA elicits potent prophylactic and therapeutic antitumoral immunity. *Cancer Research*, **70**(22), 9031–9040.

[15] Alberer, M, Gnad-Vogt, U, Hong, HS, Mehr, KT, Backert, L, Finak, G, Gottardo, R, Bica, MA, Garofano, A, Koch, SD, Fotin-Mleczek, M, Hoerr, I, Clemens, R & von Sonnenburg, F (2017). Safety and immunogenicity of a mRNA rabies vaccine in healthy adults: an open-label, non-randomised, prospective, first-in-human phase 1 clinical trial. *The Lancet*, **390**(10101), 1511–1520.

[16] Leal, L, Guardo, AC, Morón-López, S, Salgado, M, Mothe, B, Heirman, C, Pannus, P, Vanham, G, van den Ham, HJ, Gruters, R, Andeweg, A, van Meirvenne, S, Pich, J, Arnaiz, JA, Gatell, JM, Brander, C, Thielemans, K, Martínez-Picado, J, Plana, M & García, F (2018). Phase I clinical trial of an intranodally administered mRNA-based therapeutic vaccine against HIV-1 infection. *AIDS*, **32**(17), 2533–2545.

[17] de Jong, W, Aerts, J, Allard, S, Brander, C, Buyze, J, Florence, E, van Gorp, E, Vanham, G, Leal, L, Mothe, B, Thielemans, K, Plana, M, Garcia, F & Gruters, R (2019). Correction to: iHIVARNA phase iIa, a randomized, placebo-controlled, double-blinded trial to evaluate the safety and immunogenicity of iHIVARNA-01 in chronically HIV-infected patients under stable combined antiretroviral therapy. *Trials*, **20**(1), 721.

[18] Aliprantis, AO, Shaw, CA, Griffin, P, Farinola, N, Railkar, RA, Cao, X, Liu, W, Sachs, JR, Swenson, CJ, Lee, H, Cox, KS, Spellman, DS, Winstead, CJ, Smolenov, I, Lai, E, Zaks, T, Espeseth, AS & Panther, L (2020). A phase 1, randomized, placebo-controlled study to evaluate the safety and immunogenicity of an mRNA-based RSV prefusion F protein vaccine in healthy younger and older adults. *Human Vaccines & Immunotherapeutics*, **17**(5), 1248–1261.

[19] Egan, KP, Hook, LM, Naughton, A, Pardi, N, Awasthi, S, Cohen, GH, Weissman, D & Friedman, HM (2020). An HSV-2 nucleoside-modified mRNA genital herpes vaccine containing glycoproteins gC, gD, and gE protects mice against HSV-1 genital lesions and latent infection. *PLOS Pathogens*, **16**(7), e1008795.

[20] Roth, C, Cantaert, T, Colas, C, Prot, M, Casadémont, I, Levillayer, L, Thalmensi, J, Langlade-Demoyen, P, Gerke, C, Bahl, K, Ciaramella, G, Simon-Loriere, E & Sakuntabhai, A (2019). A modified mRNA vaccine targeting immunodominant ns epitopes protects against dengue virus infection in HLA class I transgenic mice. *Frontiers in Immunology*, **10**, 1424.

[21] Lo, MK, Spengler, JR, Welch, SR, Harmon, JR, Coleman-McCray, JD, Scholte, FEM, Shrivastava-Ranjan, P, Montgomery, JM, Nichol, ST, Weissman, D & Spiropoulou, CF (2019). Evaluation of a single-dose nucleoside-modified messenger RNA vaccine encoding hendra virus-soluble glycoprotein against lethal Nipah virus challenge in Syrian hamsters. *The Journal of Infectious Diseases*, **221**(Supplement_4), S493–S498.

[22] Kreiter, S, Selmi, A, Diken, M, Sebastian, M, Osterloh, P, Schild, H, Huber, C, Türeci, Z & Sahin, U (2007). Increased antigen presentation efficiency by coupling antigens to MHC Class I trafficking signals. *The Journal of Immunology*, **180**(1), 309–318.

[23] Britten, CM, Singh-Jasuja, H, Flamion, B, Hoos, A, Huber, C, Kallen, KJ, Khleif, SN, Kreiter, S, Nielsen, M, Rammensee, HG, Sahin, U, Hinz, T & Kalinke, U (2013). The regulatory landscape for actively personalized cancer immunotherapies. *Nature Biotechnology*, **31**(10), 880–882.

[24] Kranz, LM, *et al.* (2016). Systemic RNA delivery to dendritic cells exploits antiviral defence for cancer immunotherapy. *Nature*, **534**(7607), 396–401.

[25] Sahin, U, *et al.* (2017). Personalized RNA mutanome vaccines mobilize poly-specific therapeutic immunity against cancer. *Nature*, **547**(7662), 222–226.

[26] Skowronski, DM & De Serres, G (2021). Safety and efficacy of the BNT162b2 mRNA Covid-19 vaccine. *New England Journal of Medicine*, **384**(16), 1576–1578.

[27] Wetsman, N (2022, August 26). Moderna is suing Pfizer over its coronavirus vaccine. *The Verge*. https://www.theverge.com/2022/8/26/23323082/moderna-lawsuit-pfizer-mrna-vaccine-patent.

[28] Li, YD, Chi, WY, Su, JH, Ferrall, L, Hung, CF & Wu, TC (2020). Coronavirus vaccine development: from SARS and MERS to COVID-19. *Journal of Biomedical Science*, **27**(1), 104.

[29] Wu, A, Peng, Y, Huang, B, Ding, X, Wang, X, Niu, P, Meng, J, Zhu, Z, Zhang, Z, Wang, J, Sheng, J, Quan, L, Xia, Z, Tan, W, Cheng, G & Jiang, T (2020). Genome composition and divergence of the novel coronavirus (2019-nCoV) originating in China. *Cell Host & Microbe*, **27**(3), 325–328.

[30] Pardi, N, Hogan, MJ, Porter, FW & Weissman, D (2018). mRNA vaccines — a new era in vaccinology. *Nature Reviews Drug Discovery*, **17**(4), 261–279.

[31] Rosa, SS, Prazeres, DM, Azevedo, AM & Marques, MP (2021). mRNA vaccines manufacturing: challenges and bottlenecks. *Vaccine*, **39**(16), 2190–2200.

[32] Skowronski, DM & De Serres, G (2021). Safety and efficacy of the BNT162b2 mRNA Covid-19 vaccine. *New England Journal of Medicine*, **384**(16), 1576–1578.

[33] Vogel, AB, Lambert, L, Kinnear, E, Busse, D, Erbar, S, Reuter, KC, Wicke, L, Perkovic, M, Beissert, T, Haas, H, Reece, ST, Sahin, U & Tregoning, JS (2018). Self-amplifying RNA vaccines give equivalent protection against influenza to mRNA vaccines but at much lower doses. *Molecular Therapy*, **26**(2), 446–455.

[34] Pollock, KM, *et al.* (2022). Safety and immunogenicity of a self-amplifying RNA vaccine against COVID-19: COVAC1, a phase I, dose-ranging trial. *eClinicalMedicine*, **44**, 101262.

https://doi.org/10.1142/9789811262821_0004

Chapter

4

Leveraging COVID-19 Diagnostics to Confront Both Epidemic and Endemic Diseases

By Anne Hoppe, Aurelia Vessiere, and Daniel G Bausch

Summary

Diagnosis is a fundamental component of patient care and surveillance and a major driver of economic and health outcomes across health systems. However, the importance of timely access to diagnostics remains under-recognised, causing diagnostics to be critically underfunded and the weakest link in the care cascade comprising screening, diagnosis, treatment, and control. The COVID-19 pandemic further exposed fundamental gaps around diagnostics in the care cascade and made clear how profoundly a lack of diagnostics can affect patients, providers, communities, and economies. Here, we first discuss some of the key lessons from the COVID-19 pandemic before laying out a cohesive plan for a better diagnostics ecosystem, based on those learnings, to prevent future pandemics. Experience from the COVID-19 pandemic and other outbreaks and recent technological advances in diagnostics and digital tools bode well not only for the future of pandemic preparedness but also for making major inroads in closing the global diagnostics gap for common endemic diseases seen every day. However, formidable organisational, logistical, and financial obstacles must be overcome. The future can look bright if the political will is there.

Introduction

Diagnosis is a fundamental component of patient care and surveillance and a major driver of economic and health outcomes across health systems. Diagnostics are also one of three core pillars of global health security and universal health coverage, alongside vaccinations and therapeutics. However, the importance of timely access to accurate diagnostics remains under-recognised, causing diagnostics to be critically underfunded and the weakest link in the care cascade comprising screening, diagnosis, treatment, and control. The 2021 Lancet Commission on Diagnostics [1] estimates that 47% of the global population has little to no access to essential diagnostics. The lack of affordable and effective diagnostics is a life-threatening crisis for billions of people worldwide, posing a startling and significant barrier to addressing public health priorities.

Rapidly providing accurate diagnosis during epidemics and pandemics requires a number of enabling factors (Figure 4.1). The COVID-19 pandemic further exposed fundamental gaps around diagnostics in the care cascade and made clear how profoundly a lack of diagnostics can affect patients, providers, communities, and economies. Here, we first discuss some of the key lessons (Table 4.1) regarding diagnostics from the COVID-19 pandemic before laying out essential points for diagnostics, based on those lessons, to confront both epidemic and endemic diseases.

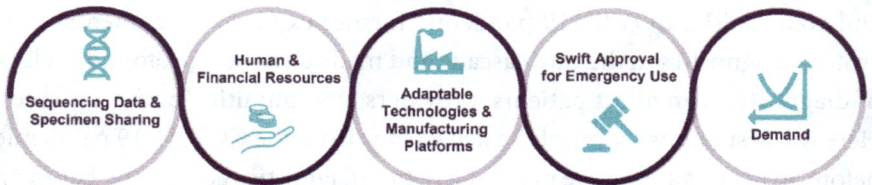

Figure 4.1   Factors enabling the rapid development of diagnostics during a pandemic.

What have we Learned about Diagnostics from the COVID-19 Pandemic?

The COVID-19 pandemic showed that we have the technological capacity to rapidly develop and scale up diagnostics for a newly emerged pathogen

Table 4.1 Key lessons learned during the COVID-19 pandemic.

1. The deployment of diagnostics across diverse geographies and settings is essential for ensuring swift and accurate identification of pathogens and preventing the spread of infectious diseases.
2. Coordinated, international partnerships are crucial for equitable access to diagnostics, treatments, and vaccines.
3. Existing diagnostic kits and platforms can be swiftly adapted to new pathogens if there are sufficient incentives and demand to do so.
4. Easily adaptable manufacturing platforms need to be available worldwide to ensure more equitable global access.
5. Testing strategies must be context-specific and coupled with extensive community engagement.
6. The integration of digital tools facilitates patient management, contact tracing, and surveillance.
7. Surveillance for epidemic-prone diseases must be integrated into surveillance for endemic diseases.

when the political will is there. Through national COVID-19 response programmes and coordinated global efforts like the Access to COVID-19 Tools (ACT) Accelerator [2, 3], launched by the WHO and partners in April 2020, the health community supported the fastest, most coordinated global effort in history to apply testing to a major pandemic. As a result, diagnostics such as nucleic acid amplification tests (NAATs) and antigen rapid diagnostic tests (Ag-RDTs) were rapidly developed and among the first tools deployed in the COVID-19 response (Figure 4.2), with genomic sequencing later playing a crucial role as the importance of tracking virus evolution became clear. Serologic tests were also eventually developed.

The success in development and scaling of SARS-CoV-2 diagnostics can be attributed to numerous factors, including early publicly available full-length sequences of SARS-CoV-2 [4]; collaboration between clinicians, academia, and industry to share data and biomaterial from patients with COVID-19 [5]; ability and readiness to divert expertise and public funding to the pandemic [3]; adaptability of technologies and manufacturing platforms that were already available for other diseases; swift authorisations for emergency use, and high demand from governments, increasing manufacturing capacity and capabilities, and reducing costs, leading eventually to increased access to tests in low- and middle-income countries (LMICs) [6].

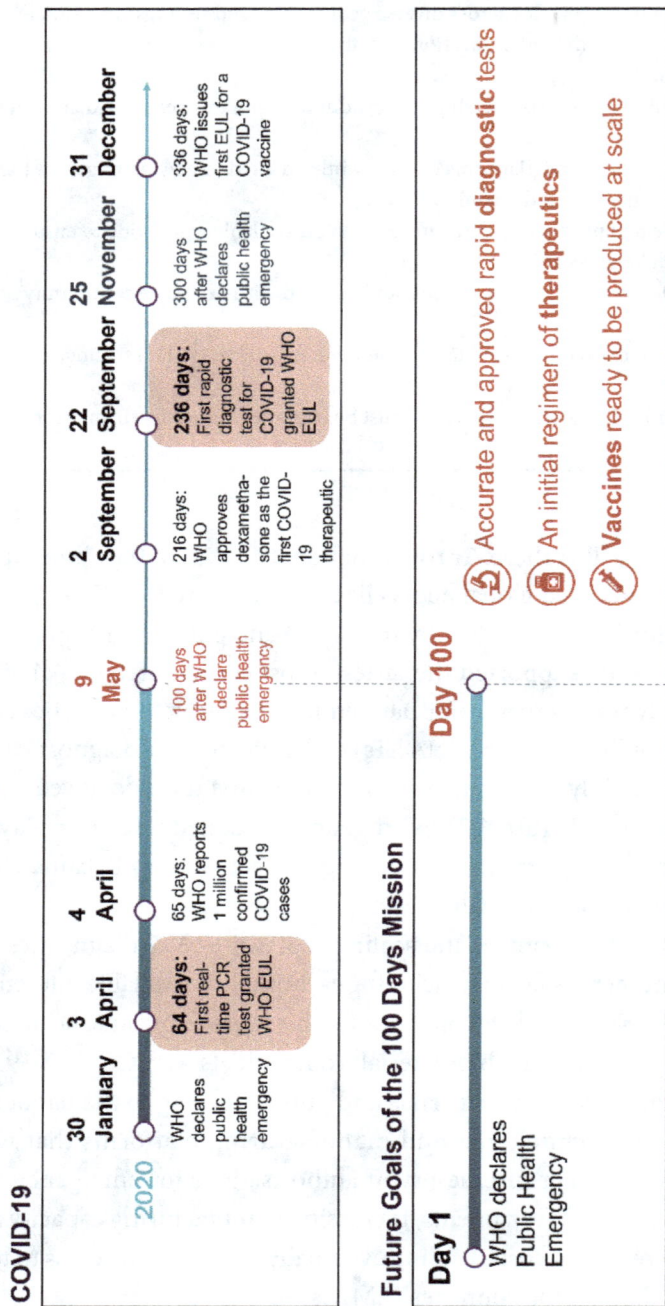

COVID-19

2020

30 January — WHO declares public health emergency

3 April — **64 days:** First real-time PCR test granted WHO EUL

4 April — 65 days: WHO reports 1 million confirmed COVID-19 cases

9 May — 100 days after WHO declare public health emergency

2 September — 216 days: WHO approves dexamethasone as the first COVID-19 therapeutic

22 September — **236 days:** First rapid diagnostic test for COVID-19 granted WHO EUL

25 November — 300 days after WHO declares public health emergency

31 December — 336 days: WHO issues first EUL for a COVID-19 vaccine

Future Goals of the 100 Days Mission

Day 1 — WHO declares Public Health Emergency

Day 100

- Accurate and approved rapid **diagnostic** tests
- An initial regimen of **therapeutics**
- **Vaccines** ready to be produced at scale

EUL: emergency use listing procedure; PCR: polymerase chain reaction; WHO: World Health Organization

Figure 4.2   Timeline of key developments of medical counter measures in the first year of the COVID-19 pandemic (top panel) and ambitions for the 100 Days Mission (bottom panel).

Nucleic Acid Amplification Tests

On 17 January 2022, 13 days before the COVID-19 outbreak was declared a public health emergency of international concern (PHEIC), WHO issued their first interim guidance to laboratories, which called for use of pan-coronavirus NAATs, with subsequent sequencing of non-conserved regions of amplicons to confirm SARS-CoV-2 [7]. Polymerase chain reaction tests for SARS-CoV-2 became available for limited use in laboratories eight days after the PHEIC was declared, and were subsequently authorised and available for scaled-up testing in major health centres within 64 days following the declaration. Since then, over 650 NAATs have been developed and are commercially available [6].

While NAATs are generally highly sensitive and considered the gold standard for detecting SARS-CoV-2, and availability of the platform has increased over the past decade, there are still substantial barriers to widespread NAAT use, including costs for equipment and reagents, the requirement for trained laboratory technicians, and issues of equipment maintenance and quality control. The United States Centers for Disease Control and Prevention (CDC) estimates the cost of a polymerase chain reaction test for SARS-CoV-2 to be USD 75–100 [8]. Furthermore, most NAATs require an uninterrupted power supply, and diagnosis usually takes several hours to days, which hampers swift identification of infected individuals. This delay may impede the utility of NAATs from the perspectives of both public health (*i.e.*, rapidly identifying infected persons to take steps to prevent transmission) and patient management (*i.e.*, delaying diagnosis for appropriate triage and clinical management).

Antigen Rapid Diagnostic Tests

In light of the limitations of NAATs, public health authorities and manufacturers pursued the development of SARS-CoV-2 Ag-RDTs. Ag-RDTs are usually relatively inexpensive, easy to use, and provide results within 30 minutes, as evidenced by their frequent use for detection of malaria in LMICs since the early 1990s [9]. Since they do not require a cold chain for transport or storage, RDTs can be easily deployed in a variety of settings. However, relative to NAATs, RDT technology is harder to adapt to new pathogens; the first SARS-CoV-2 Ag-RDTs were only available 236 days after the COVID-19

PHEIC declaration. At least 39 Ag-RDTs have since been authorised for use by WHO [6]. The key limitation of Ag-RDTs is their lower sensitivity, leading the CDC to recommend repeat testing (after 48 hours or more) or follow-up NAAT to confirm a negative Ag-RTD result [8].

Genomic Sequencing

As the pandemic progressed, there was increasing recognition of the risk of emergence of potentially dangerous new SARS-CoV-2 variants, highlighting the need for genomic sequencing to understand and keep to stay ahead of the evolving virus, to ensure that existing diagnostics, vaccines, and therapeutics (especially those based on molecular approaches) were still effective [10, 11]. Systematic genomic sequencing of a subset of SARS-CoV-2 specimens became the goal, and eventually the norm, in most high-income countries, with budding capacity in many LMICs as well; South Africa's and Botswana's genomic surveillance programmes were able to rapidly alert the world to the existence of the dangerous SARS-CoV-2 Omicron variant [12, 13]. The existence of corresponding metadata (*i.e.*, clinical and epidemiological information) is essential to interpret the significance of the sequence data. There is also often the need for follow-up laboratory investigations to associate phenotypic characteristics with genotype.

Serology

Serologic tests for SARS-CoV-2 antibody were developed later in the pandemic and helped assess the level of population exposure to virus in many countries and regions. However, there were, and remain, major problems with standardisation and interpretation of serologic tests; because the correlates of protection for COVID-19 remain poorly defined, the presence of antibody does not necessarily confirm immunity, nor the lack of it confirm susceptibility. Measures of cellular immunity can help with interpretation, but are more difficult to assess.

Challenges

While the COVID-19 pandemic heightened awareness of the crucial role of diagnostics in healthcare and control measures, diagnostics gaps and challenges persist for both COVID-19 and the broad range of non-COVID-19 health threats. Assay development for SARS-CoV-2 was initially hindered due to slow access to samples and reference material, lack of clear product requirements, and insufficient regulatory harmonisation. The market was underprepared, with an initial lack of demand and supportive policies for affordable, fast, and accurate diagnostics prior to the COVID-19 pandemic and limited evidence to inform policy and build manufacturing capacity. Although costs for Ag-RDTs eventually came down, and supply increased, access to accurate tests in LMICs and integration into surveillance networks remained fundamental issues during the pandemic [14, 15].

What Should we do to Prevent Future Pandemics?

The 100 Days Mission: The Marathon Before the Sprint

Looking forwards, it is important to identify and implement effective new approaches to close the diagnostic gap, saving lives, and enhancing equitable provision of healthcare. In June 2021, the G7 countries met and called for a "100 Days Mission to Respond to Future Pandemic Threats" in which the world would develop the capacity to produce the key tools—diagnostics, vaccines, and therapeutics—to respond within 100 days after WHO declaration of a major infectious disease event (Figure 4.2) [16]. FIND (Geneva, Switzerland), in collaboration with the Coalition for Epidemic Preparedness Innovations (Oslo, Norway) and other partners, has developed an 11-step programme to achieve this goal with regard to diagnostics (Figure 4.3). Below we elaborate on some key components crucial to success.

Accelerate Product Research and Development

Success in the 100 Days Mission will require a range of diagnostic tools to be employed across the spectrum of care settings, from RDTs that an individual can use at home or in the workplace, to genomic sequencing capacity at national or regional reference centers. The COVID-19 pandemic has brought about the routinisation of existing platforms, such as RDTs, and many promising products are emerging onto the market. Of particular promise are molecular multiplex assays that are easy to use and sufficiently robust and inexpensive to allow for use even in LMICs. Integration into routine use at

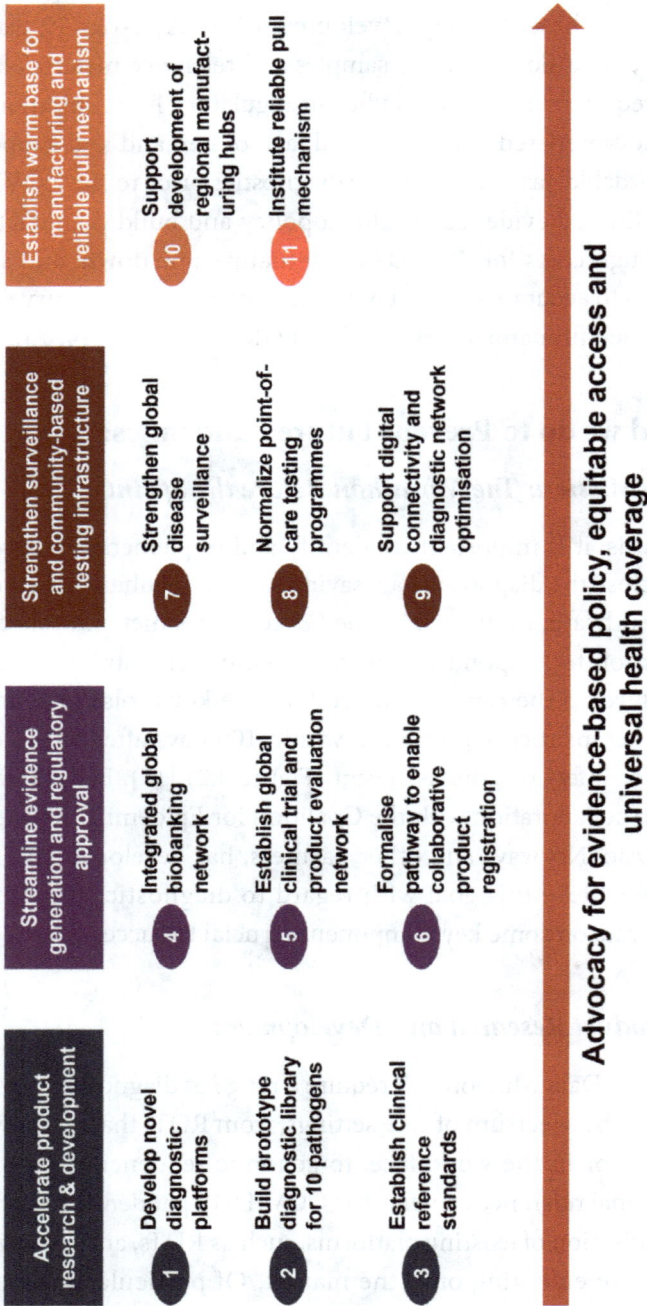

Figure 4.3   The FIND 5-year initiative to enable the 100 Days Mission for diagnostics.

the primary care level, supported by appropriate training of healthcare workers and implementation of systems for remote quality control through digital technologies, could be game changing. Still more advanced technologies and novel diagnostic platforms are on the horizon, many close to being ready for use (Figure 4.4).

Advancing these tools requires more than simply competent laboratories and scientists. Clinical reference standards must be established to create common goals and facilitate technology transfer among industry and academic partners engaged in research and development (R&D). To adapt innovative products to outbreak prevention, there must be agreement on the first targets or "priority pathogens" that are deemed outbreak-prone, accounting also for "pathogen X", *i.e.*, a truly novel emerging agent. The prioritisation list should take into account not only the likelihood of human infection with a given pathogen but also the potential impact of an outbreak (disease severity, social, economic and cultural impact, political impact and effects on global health security). Various priority pathogen lists have been emitted from a host of different agencies, but there is not yet universal agreement. Nevertheless, at the time of this writing, WHO is organising a meeting to arrive at a consensus [17]. Although the focus is overwhelmingly and appropriately on viruses,

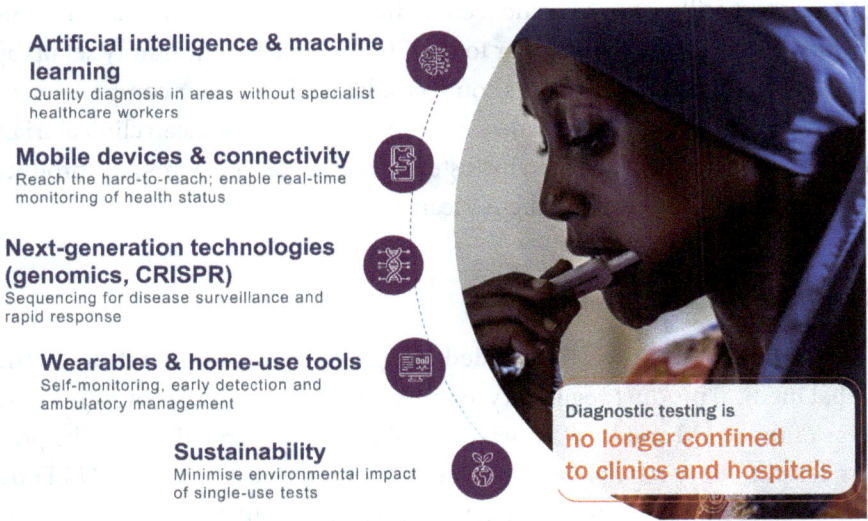

Artificial intelligence & machine learning
Quality diagnosis in areas without specialist healthcare workers

Mobile devices & connectivity
Reach the hard-to-reach; enable real-time monitoring of health status

Next-generation technologies (genomics, CRISPR)
Sequencing for disease surveillance and rapid response

Wearables & home-use tools
Self-monitoring, early detection and ambulatory management

Sustainability
Minimise environmental impact of single-use tests

Diagnostic testing is
no longer confined
to clinics and hospitals

Figure 4.4 Innovative and potential game-changing diagnostic technologies on the horizon, accelerated in part by the COVID-19 pandemic.

the threat of antimicrobially resistant bacteria should not be forgotten. The generally agreed-upon approach is to build prototype diagnostic libraries for priority pathogens, with the belief that diagnostics manufacturers will be able to rapidly pivot to similar pathogens from the same virus family that might cause an outbreak, even if it is not the exact pathogen for which the diagnostic test was developed.

R&D of diagnostics for outbreak-prone pathogens requires access to biomaterial, including both pathogen isolates and clinical material (*e.g.*, blood, serum, nasopharyngeal swabs), both before and during an outbreak. Infrastructure and accords for biobanking and equitable sharing of biomaterial across public and private sector partners will be essential. These must include guarantees that countries who share biomaterial will also share in the benefits, *i.e.*, the diagnostics produced. Creating a global framework for rapid clinical evaluation of new diagnostics and testing algorithms will also be essential.

During the COVID-19 pandemic, a large network of partners was built with capabilities in biobanking and product evaluation of diagnostics both in the laboratory and the field. We must now capitalise on this network by creating and maintaining a community of stakeholders with the right expertise and capacities. The matter is far from simple, however, considering the difficulty in not only predicting what will be the next pathogen to emerge but also where it will occur, as evidenced by the recent global outbreak of monkeypox. A model which is similar to the Clinical Trials Community set up by the African Academy of Sciences could be adapted [18]. Their comprehensive and transparent database provides real-time visibility of African clinical trials sites and their capabilities, thereby fostering collaborations across the product development ecosystem and the African continent.

Regulatory Harmonisation

The COVID-19 pandemic revealed the piecemeal fragmentation of the global medical product regulatory architecture, with rapid approvals in some areas of the world and lengthy delays in others. In the United States, the process for obtaining regulatory approvals is harmonised through the US Food and Drug Administration, but such overarching regulatory authorities are not present in all the world's regions. In Europe, the process for obtaining exceptional-use regulatory approvals is not harmonised, with authorisation occurring via individual member state processes. Efforts are under way to improve harmonisation across Africa through the recently created African Medicines Agency [19] and related efforts of the African Medical Devices Forum. However, further optimisations are needed to ensure swift availability of safe and effective diagnostics in all settings across the globe. This should include processes for rapid development of Target Product Profiles and technical specifications around different use cases, timely and transparent publication of patient information and product evaluation studies to fast-track Exceptional Use Authorisations, and digitally enabled post-market surveillance/follow-up systems. Investment in training will be required to scale up regional and global regulatory capacity and capability.

Bringing Diagnostics Closer to the Patient, Healthcare Provider, and Community — the Right Tools to the Right People

Diagnostic testing has traditionally required a visit to a healthcare professional or laboratory. However, there are many barriers to access and to this approach, including lack of healthcare coverage, transportation costs, loss of income due to the time required to seek care, and long waiting times for results (which may lead to enhanced transmission due to delays in disease recognition and implementation of infection prevention and control measures). For example, in Africa almost 80% of individuals are not paid employees and therefore do not receive a regular wage but rather are dependent on daily income [20]. Furthermore, especially in resource-limited communities, only severely symptomatic individuals may be likely to seek diagnosis and medical care. Even when patients do have access to care, in many LMICs diagnostic test availability at the primary healthcare level is often woefully lacking [1, 21].

Newer technologies such as RDTs, for which familiarity has now become almost universal, present an opportunity for a drastic restructuring of the diagnostics landscape, placing rapidly actionable evidence in the hands of the healthcare provider or even individual patient through point-of-care or near point-of-care testing (Figure 4.5). In addition, RDTs hold enormous potential for locally adapted community-based and community-driven testing and intervention strategies, including in schools, markets, and at borders and transport hubs. However, care must be taken to avoid unintended negative consequences. For example, RDT use resulting in strictly enforced home- or facility-based isolation of people testing positive to prevent transmission may

Pre-COVID-19

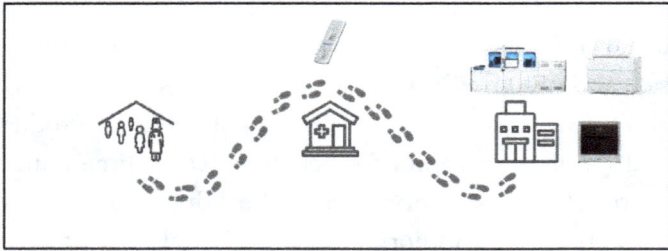

AT HOME   PRIMARY   HOSPITAL /
                 CARE   LABORATORY

Post-COVID-19 Innovation

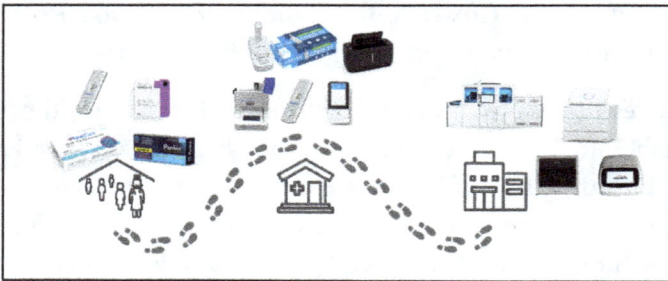

Figure 4.5   COVID-19 driven innovation: connected diagnostics and interoperable systems for data management, data aggregation, and data sharing for surveillance. *Images of specific assays are included for illustrative purposes and do not constitute an endorsement.*

be effective in the short term, but in the long term could provoke resistance to getting tested. Another concern is the difficulty of collecting surveillance data when testing is decentralised. While a legitimate concern, this should not be a barrier to the rapid provision of actionable diagnosis into the hands of the individual patient and the healthcare provider. Sentinel surveillance approaches and integration of novel digital tools (see Figure 4.5) may ultimately allow the best of both worlds.

Strengthening Global Disease Surveillance

Surveillance of infectious diseases has been fragmented during the COVID-19 pandemic due to the diversion of resources and profound disruption of health systems. COVID-19 surveillance was generally ad hoc and standalone, not integrated into surveillance for other respiratory diseases, such as influenza. Although there is much interest in developing them, integrated cost-effective, context-specific surveillance systems are yet to be established. Nevertheless, the burgeoning repertoire of diagnostic tools — from RDTs to genomic sequencing — holds the promise of advanced event- and indicator-based surveillance spanning the gamut of levels of care that could be transformative in early warning and response. It will be important to place the right tools in the right settings, *e.g.*, RDTs to the individual at home, simple multiplex diagnostics at the primary and secondary care levels, increasing to more advanced diagnostic platforms such as blood culture and next-generation sequencing at the tertiary care level and at reference centres. There must be clear linkages and algorithms for when to test at higher levels of the healthcare system, with results digitally connected to centralised databases designed for rapid analysis and keyed to specific actions in response [15].

While the focus is often understandably on pathogens of epidemic potential, it is essential that surveillance for these pathogens be systematically integrated into surveillance for everyday endemic diseases. Some success has been noted for integration of SARS-CoV-2 testing into existing surveillance activities for endemic diseases such as malaria [22]. Experience has shown that parallel vertical approaches to emerging disease surveillance are unlikely to be sustainable. While outbreaks may be generally increasing in incidence, emergence of any given epidemic-prone pathogen, usually zoonotic, continues to be a rare event. For example, despite the upheaval and loss of life it causes, there have been less than 40 recorded primary introductions (*i.e.*, human infection from a natural reservoir) of Ebola virus into humans since the virus was discovered in 1976. It is essential to move beyond traditional binary approaches, *e.g.*, diagnostics that render a positive or negative result for only a single pathogen, with a negative test being of little use to the still sick patient or the field team investigating an outbreak. In the long term, only approaches that show regular actionable value to the patient, healthcare provider, and local and national governments will continue to be practiced and funded.

Manufacturing and Supply Chains

While over 1,000 assays to detect SARS-CoV-2 infection have been marketed, nearly all are manufactured in high- or middle-income countries in

Asia, Europe, or North America (Figure 4.6) [6]. To be prepared for the next pandemic, it will be crucial to develop a much broader and more equitable manufacturing base through the development of regional manufacturing hubs, especially in LMICs, with novel, nimble, and adaptable diagnostic platforms that can ensure production and maintenance of supply on a local and regional level. It is also essential to build sufficient capacity so that production of diagnostics during an outbreak does not infringe on continued production of routine diagnostics, impeding diagnosis and care for endemic diseases. Beyond issues of supply, broadening the global base of manufacturing capacity will also enable innovative contributions to R&D from more partners, especially those in LMICs.

Creative thinking and approaches will be necessary to ensure economic viability and sustainability of this new manufacturing and pipeline landscape, which will presumably comprise a larger number of smaller facilities. While pandemics and large epidemics may create a viable and sustainable commercial demand, diagnostics for epidemic-prone diseases that are rarely seen or cause problems on a more restricted local or regional scale, especially in LMICs, are unlikely to be addressed through traditional for-profit commercial approaches. Rather, considerations must be made for advance volume commitments, preferential pricing, and agreements on technology transfer and intellectual property. Solutions will ideally be based on more nimble and economically efficient "pull systems" that initiate production as a reaction to present demand (as opposed to more wasteful "push systems" in which production is initiated independently of demand).

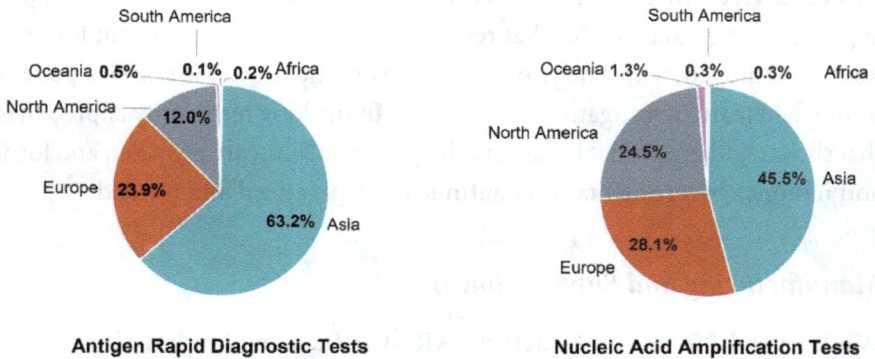

Figure 4.6   Geographic distribution of manufacturing sites for SARS-CoV-2 diagnostics.

Digital Tools

Recent decades have seen incredible advances in digital technologies, which have been increasingly applied to health, a process accelerated by the COVID-19 pandemic. Digital tools have been used to support patient management by interlinking demographic, clinical, and laboratory data and to facilitate monitoring of patient outcomes; for remote quality assurance and quality control of tests, thereby reducing the costs of in-field deployment of diagnostics; to strengthen case detection and contact tracing; and to ensure data capture and aggregation at sub-district, district, and country levels, thereby strengthening both localised and central surveillance activities [23]. To help health systems monitor and prepare for pandemics at the frontlines of service delivery, digital tools can support decentralisation of diagnosis, including delivery of point-of-care testing at the community level, in several ways: by conducting real-time data capture and transmission to facilitate monitoring and epidemiological surveillance; providing clinical guidance such as screening algorithms to determine which patients to prioritise for testing [24]; improving linkage to care [25]; and facilitating more efficient use of resources [26].

However, many challenges remain to maximise the impact of these powerful digital tools, including harmonising diverse data capture systems and programmes and integrating approaches to avoid many cumbersome vertical systems relevant only to a single or few diseases. Interoperability of digital systems is key to supporting health programmes in using the data being generated from different efforts in a cohesive and comprehensible manner for pandemic preparedness, while reuse of existing digital tools can help ensure that fragmentation of digital investments and efforts is minimised. The WHO digital health atlas and other such resources can be leveraged by partners interested in this field as a starting point to map out available tools and projects in countries [27].

Equity and Access

While inequity in the distribution of COVID-19 vaccines was well publicised, there were also inequities with regards to diagnostics, especially early in the pandemic, when supplies of NAAT reagents and first-generation test kits were still limited. Inequitable access was exacerbated by the impact of lockdowns and travel restrictions on global supply pipelines, with LMICs being especially vulnerable. Even as supply increased, insufficient purchasing power in LMICs put them last in line. For instance, large orders of Ag-RDTs placed by the United States in early 2022 decreased their availability in Africa, South America, and the Caribbean [personal communication].

While advocating for more equitable access to medical countermeasures, including diagnostics, is always warranted, human nature to protect one's own and political pressures on national leaders to prioritise local and national populations make it unlikely that equity will be achieved on moral grounds alone. Rather, access must be ensured through systematically building equity into health and preparedness systems in advance. This means creating more globally distributed manufacturing bases and supply pipelines, advance purchase agreements, and plans to secure supply pipelines to ensure equitable access when emergencies arrive. The COVID-19 pandemic has taught us how connected our planet is. Thus, ensuring global access is not only a compelling moral argument but also a strategic one — no one is safe until everyone is safe.

Lastly, and perhaps most importantly, we must enhance our advocacy for universal health coverage, which underpins virtually everything in pandemic preparedness. A sick person who does not have access to care does not get evaluated, diagnosed, or treated. Neither the individual nor the public health system know what disease they might have. With no diagnosis, there is no possibility to respond on either the individual (*i.e.*, treating the patient) or population (*i.e.*, implementing disease prevention measures) levels.

Advocating for Evidence-Based Policy

Evidence-based policymaking is essential to build trust within communities, and better engagement with populations at risk will improve both surveillance and intervention strategies. It was apparent during the COVID-19 pandemic that it is not sufficient for safe and effective diagnostics to be available; local and global policies often determine how diagnostics are deployed and hence how effective they are in leading to appropriate clinical care and prevention of transmission [28]. During the pandemic, policymakers frequently had to make decisions before conclusive scientific evidence that supported their policies was available. Some global leaders set policy that ignored or was even in direct conflict with existing evidence, affecting the credibility of both policymakers and scientists. The scientific community must continue to be and must grow further as a voice advocating evidence-based policy.

Financing

Of course, sufficient funding is essential to make the 100 Days Mission a reality — a goal challenged by fading memories once an epidemic or pandemic begins to wane, the many competing global needs, and the current or impending global economic recession, among many other factors. The World Bank has recently created a Pandemic Fund to "finance critical investments to strengthen pandemic prevention, preparedness, and response capacities at national, regional, and global levels, with a focus on low- and middle-income countries" [29]. While laudable, the mechanism for dispersion of funds remains to be determined, and there are concerns over the relatively small sum for such an ambitious agenda (USD 1.4 billion at the time of writing) and that this mechanism may potentially compete with or draw funds away from funding for other public health organisations and programmes.

An International Diagnostic Alliance: Working Together for a Better Diagnostics Ecosystem

While there are many successes to cite from the COVID-19 response, and reasons for optimism for future pandemic preparedness, there are also many challenges. A major one is fragmentation of the diagnostics ecosystem. While there is a plethora of public and private sector partners with good intentions, to date there is no convening body to set a common course and foster collaboration and synergies across stakeholders. Success will require a multisectoral approach involving, among others, natural and social scientists, manufacturers, healthcare and public health professionals, policymakers, community leaders, and communities. While the ACT Accelerator undoubtedly contributed to many successes and may serve as a starting template, not all LMIC partners felt well represented in that mechanism.

The 2021 Lancet Commission on Diagnostics [1] identified challenges and recommended establishing a global Alliance for Diagnostics to coordinate, support, monitor, and ensure accountability of diagnostic priorities. Discussions between various partners are underway to create such an alliance. In addition, a proposal has been submitted for a World Health Assembly Resolution on essential diagnostics capacity, highlighting the need for an end-to-end approach to addressing diagnostic needs and priorities. Experience from the COVID-19 pandemic and other outbreaks, as well as recent technological advances in diagnostics and digital tools, bode well for the future not only of pandemic preparedness but also for making major inroads in closing the global diagnostics gap for common endemic diseases seen every day. However, formidable organisational, logistical, and financial obstacles must be overcome. The future can look bright if the political will is there.

Acknowledgements

The authors thank Rigveda Kadam and Robyn Meurant for technical input.

References

[1] Fleming, KA, Horton, S, Wilson, ML, Atun, R, DeStigter, K, Flanigan, J, Sayed, S, Adam, P, Aguilar, B, Andronikou, S, Boehme, C, Cherniak, W, Cheung, ANY, Dahn, B, Donoso-Bach, L, Douglas, T, Garcia, P, Hussain, S, Hari, S Iyer, HS, Kohli, M, Labrique, AB, Looi, L-M, Meara, JG, Nkengasong, J, Pai, M, Pool, K-L, Ramaiya, K, Schroeder, L, Shah, D, Sullivan, R, Tan, B-S & Walia, K (2001). The Lancet Commission on diagnostics: transforming access to diagnostics. *Lancet*, **398**, 1997–2050.

[2] The Access to COVID-19 Tools (ACT) Accelerator (n.d.). *WHO*. https://www.who.int/initiatives/act-accelerator.

[3] ACT Accelerator — Access to COVID-19 Tools (n.d.). *WHO*. https://www.act-a.org/diagnostics.

[4] Novel 2019 coronavirus genoma (n.d.). *Virological*. http://virological.org/t/novel-2019-coronavirus-genome/319.

[5] Harrison, PW, Rodrigo Lopez, R, Rahman, N, Allen, SG, Aslam, R, Buso, N, Cummins, C, Fathy, Y, Felix, E, Glont, M, Jayathilaka, S, Kadam, S, Kumar, M, Lauer, KB, Malhotra, G, Mosaku, A, Edbali, O, Park, YM, Parton, A, Pearce, M, Pena, JFE, Rossetto, J, Russell, C, Selvakumar, S, Sitja, XP, Sokolov, A, Thorne, R, Ventouratou, M, Walter, P, Yordanova, G, Zadissa, A, Cochrane, G, Blomberg, N & Apweiler, R (2021). The COVID-19 data portal: accelerating SARS-CoV-2 and COVID-19 research through rapid open access data sharing. *Nucleic Acids Research*, **49**, W619–W623.

[6] FIND Test Directory (n.d.). *FIND*. https://www.finddx.org/covid-19/test-directory/.

[7] Laboratory testing for 2019 novel coronavirus (2019-nCoV) in suspected human cases (2020, March 19). *WHO*. https://www.who.int/publications/i/item/10665-331501.

[8] Guidance for antigen testing for SARS-CoV-2 for healthcare providers testing individuals in the community (2020, April 4). *U.S. Centers for Disease Control and Prevention*.

https://www.cdc.gov/coronavirus/2019-ncov/lab/resources/antigen-tests-guidelines. html#anchor_1631295313910.

[9] Thepsamarn, P, Prayoollawongsa, N, Puksupa, P, Puttoom, P, Thaidumrong, P, Wongchai, S, Doddara, J, Tantayarak, J, Buchachart, K, Wilairatana, P & Looareesuwan, S (1997). The ICT malaria Pf: a simple, rapid dipstick test for the diagnosis of Plasmodium falciparum malaria at the Thai-Myanmar border. *Southeast Asian Journal of Tropical Medicine and Public Health*, **28**, 723–726.

[10] Lind, ML, Copin, R, McCarthy, S, Coppi, A, Warner, F, Ferguson, D, Duckwall, C, Borg, R, Muenker, MC, Overton, J, Hamon, S, Zhou, A, Cummings, DAT, Ko, AI, Hamilton, JD, Schulz, W & Hitchings, MT (2022). Use of whole genome sequencing to estimate the contribution of immune evasion and waning immunity to decreasing COVID-19 vaccine effectiveness during alpha and delta variant waves. *Journal of Infectious Diseases*, in press. https://doi.org/10.1093/infdis/jiac453.

[11] Garcia-Beltran, WF, Lam, EC, St Denis, K, Nitido, AD, Garcia, ZH, Hauser, BM, Feldman, J, Pavlovic, MN, Gregory, DJ, Poznansky, MC, Sigal, A, Schmidt, AG, Iafrate, AJ, Naranbhai, V & Balazs, AB (2021). Multiple SARS-CoV-2 variants escape neutralization by vaccine-induced humoral immunity. *Cell*, **184**(9), 2372–2383.

[12] Classification of Omicron (B.1.1.529): SARS-CoV-2 variant of concern (2021, November 26). *WHO*. https://www.who.int/news/item/26-11-2021-classification-of-omicron-(b.1.1.529)-sars-cov-2-variant-of-concern.

[13] Cable, J, Fauci, A, Dowling, WE, Günther, S, Bente, DA, Yadav, PD, Madoff, LC, Wang, LF, Arora, RK, Van Kerkhove, M, Chu, MC, Jaenisch, T, Epstein, JH, Frost, SDW, Bausch, DG, Hensley, LE, Bergeron, É, Sitaras, I, Gunn, MD, Geisbert, TW, Muñoz-Fontela, C, Krammer, F, de Wit, E, Nordenfelt, P, Saphire, EO, Gilbert, SC, Corbett, KS, Branco, LM, Baize, S, van Doremalen, N, Krieger, MA, Clemens, SAC, Hesselink, R & Hartman, D (2022). Lessons from the pandemic: Responding to emerging zoonotic viral diseases-a Keystone Symposia report. *Annals of the New York Academy of Sciences*, **1518**(1), 209–225.

[14] Diagnostic testing for SARS-CoV-2 (2020, September 11). *WHO*. https://www.who.int/publications/i/item/diagnostic-testing-for-sars-cov-2.

[15] Public health surveillance for COVID-19: interim guidance (2022, July 22). *WHO*. https://www.who.int/publications/i/item/WHO-2019-nCoV-SurveillanceGuidance-2022.2.

[16] A report to the G7 by the pandemic preparedness partnership: 100 days mission to respond to future pandemic threats (2021, June 12). *G7 Summit 2021*. https://assets.publishing.service.gov.uk/government/uploads/system/uploads/attachment_data/file/992762/100_Days_Mission_to_respond_to_future_pandemic_threats__3_.pdf.

[17] WHO to identify pathogens that could cause future outbreaks and pandemics (2022, November 21). *WHO*. https://www.who.int/news/item/21-11-2022-who-to-identify-pathogens-that-could-cause-future-outbreaks-and-pandemics.

[18] Promoting clinical trials in Africa through harmonized stakeholder engagement (n.d.). *African Academy of Sciences*. https://www.aasciences.africa/aesa/programmes/clinical-trials-community#:~:text=Promoting%20Clinical%20Trials%20in%20Africa%20through%20Harmonized%20Stakeholder%20Engagement.

[19] African Medicines Regulatory Harmonization (n.d.). *Tanzania Medicines & Medical Devices Authority.* https://www.tmda.go.tz/pages/african-medicines-regulatory-harmon-isation-amrh#:~:text=The%20objective%20of%20the%20African%20Medicines%20 Regulatory%20Harmonization,of%20the%20Pharmaceutical%20Manufacturing%20 Plan%20for%20Africa%20%28PMPA%29.

[20] Wages in Africa — Recent trends in average wages, gender pay gaps and wage dispari-ties (2019, November 3). *International Labour Organization.* https://www.ilo.org/africa/ information-resources/publications/WCMS_728363/lang--en/index.htm.

[21] Yadav, H, Shah, D, Sayed, S, Horton, S & Schroeder, LF (2021). Availability of essen-tial diagnostics in ten low-income and middle-income countries: results from national health facility surveys. *Lancet Global Health,* **9**(11), e1553–e1560.

[22] Malaria Program Suriname (n.d.). *Ministerie van Volksgezondheid.* https://www. malariasuriname.com/.

[23] Guide to Global Digital Tools for COVID-19 Response (2020, October 23). *U.S. Centers for Disease Control and Prevention.* https://www.cdc.gov/coronavirus/2019-ncov/global-covid-19/compare-digital-tools.html.

[24] Zens, M, Brammertz, A, Herpich, J, Südkamp, N & Hinterseer, M. App-based tracking of self-reported COVID-19 symptoms: analysis of questionnaire data. *Journal of Medical Internet Research,* **22**(9), e21956.

[25] Pai, N, Esmail, A, Chaduri, SP, Oelofse, S, Pretorius, M, Marathe, G, Daher, J, Smallwood, M, Karatzas, N, Fadul, M, de Waal, A, Engel, N, Zwerling, AA & Dheda, K (2021). Impact of a personalised, digital, HIV self-testing app-based program on linkages and new infections in the township populations of South Africa. *BMJ Global Health,* **6**(9), e006032.

[26] Lesotho village health workers' road to a digital era (2021, April 12). *UNDP.* https://www. undp.org/lesotho/blog/lesotho-village-health-workers-road-digital-era.

[27] Digital Health Atlas (n.d.). *WHO.* https://digitalhealthatlas.org/en/-/.

[28] Jain, V, Clarke, J & Beaney, T (2022). Association between democratic governance and excess mortality during the COVID-19 pandemic: an observational study. *Journal of Epidemiology and Community Health,* **76**, 853–860.

[29] The Pandemic Fund (n.d.). *World Bank.* https://www.worldbank.org/en/programs/ financial-intermediary-fund-for-pandemic-prevention-preparedness-and-response-ppr-fif.

Chapter

5

First as Farce, Twice as Tragedy: US Exceptionalism in COVID-19 Response

By Martha Lincoln

Summary

Since the beginning of the COVID-19 pandemic, the United States has recorded epidemiological outcomes ranking far below those achieved by other wealthy democracies. In this discussion, I suggest that the nation's COVID-19 response has, under two different presidential administrations, been compromised by American exceptionalism — a cultural sense of specialness and superiority imagined as unique to the US. Both by reifying individual freedoms that are constructed as quintessentially American, and by resisting and "othering" pandemic control measures that have succeeded elsewhere in the world, US leaders and the public have committed ideologically to less effective — and often counterproductive — approaches in public health.

Introduction

From the earliest months of the COVID-19 pandemic, the United States has registered as a nearly inexplicable epidemiological outlier among the world's wealthy nations. Over two years and multiple waves of infection, its rates of per-capita coronavirus morbidity and mortality have outstripped trends in other high-income economies and disparately contributed to global totals of COVID-19 infections and deaths [1]. As early as March 2020, the US reported the highest total case count of any nation [2] — a trend that has remained essentially stable through mid-2022 [3]. Initiatives to limit community spread of the virus in many US states have been challenged by restive domestic groups as well as leaders at all levels of government. And despite the widespread availability of free and effective vaccines in the US beginning in spring 2021, rates of vaccination uptake have subsequently swiftly dropped off — showing only weak increases in response to the emergence of new variants [4]. A May 2022 report found that since the beginning of the pandemic, over half of the American population had been infected at least once [5]; just weeks later, the US was the first country in the world to record a total of 1 million deaths from COVID-19.

These dismaying outcomes have thoroughly belied prior assumptions about levels of public health capacity in the United States — which, just months before the emergence of SARS-CoV-2, was named in the 2019 Global Health Security Index (GHSI) the nation *best* prepared to contain a pandemic [6]. In its assessment of multiple indicators of national health security, the GHSI ranked the US highly for its performance across domains from "Prevention" to "Health System". Prior to the emergence of the new pathogen, Americanness was assumed — both in the GHSI rankings and elsewhere — to be synonymous with technical competence and with widely shared public acceptance of the modern health sciences and their institutions. Yet despite these confident appraisals, the early months of US response to the new virus — a response marked by inaction, shortages, nepotism, false and misleading official statements, technical missteps, anti-science sentiment, and public panic — were often compared to the experience assumed to be typical in a so-called "third-world country" [7].

Indeed, as this invocation of a shifting world order suggests, the COVID-19 pandemic and national pandemic response swiftly became sites where ideas about America and Americanness have been examined, contested, and reshaped. In the first months of 2022, US levels of per-population COVID deaths were closely comparable to casualty rates recorded in the former Yugoslavian nations, Eastern Europe, and Latin America [8]. In February 2022, the US was found to have lost a larger percentage of its population to COVID-19 than other wealthy "peer nations". Assessing the impact of the

Omicron wave in the US, the *New York Times* wrote: "The only large European countries to exceed America's COVID death rates this winter have been Russia, Ukraine, Poland, Greece and the Czech Republic" [9]. The authors of a 2022 study comparing COVID-19 mortality rates in the United States with those recorded in 20 peer OECD nations found "COVID-19 deaths per capita in the US (...) significantly exceeded those of all peer countries" during the Delta and Omicron waves [10].

Populist Leadership: A Partial Explanation

From an early moment, many analysts cited unfit national leadership as a determining factor in the inferior outcomes achieved by the US in 2020 and early 2021 [11]. This appeared persuasive not least because President Donald Trump — a leader whose paranoid style of pandemic governance openly trafficked in jingoism, xenophobia [12], and conspiracy theories [13] — appeared to be, at best, an ambivalent foe of mass infection. Though the president was aware from an early moment that the new virus consti-tuted "deadly stuff" [14], he played down this reality in public, characterising SARS-CoV-2 as causing a negligible, flu-like illness. Trump continuously endorsed anti-science sentiments via social media channels, becoming uniquely influential among world leaders in shaping public opinion about the pandemic [15]. In September 2020, the administration's indifference resulted in a super-spreader event at the White House and in Trump's own infection with the virus.

Presidential hubris in 2020 might therefore seem to represent the defining factor in the American pandemic's ruinous trajectory. Indeed, journalistic and scholarly commentary has suggested that the anti-expert and anti-scientific sentiments of "illiberal populist" or "populist nationalist" leaders — such as Trump — are associated with the inferior pandemic outcomes achieved to date by wealthy nations such as the United States, the United Kingdom, Russia, and Brazil [16, 17]. Yet the correlation between populist governance and suboptimal pandemic outcomes may need to be further nuanced. A statisti-cally based analysis found that this association is not uniform across settings: populist leaders have exerted the greatest negative impact on COVID outcomes in the world's less democratic democracies, not including the United States [18]. As such, populist governance under the Trump administration may only partially explain the nation's experience over the first two and a half years of the coronavirus pandemic.

Upon assuming office in January 2021, Trump's Democratic successor Joe Biden confronted a continuing public health emergency, as well as a crisis of public trust [19] — having promised on the campaign trail that "We're going to beat this virus" [20]. Yet the administration has proven ill equipped to achieve significant improvements in American pandemic outcomes; COVID-19 has continued to cause exceptional levels of illness, disability, and death in the US. While Biden has stridently advocated for vaccines and boosters, his administration has offered much less support for non-pharmaceutical interventions such as quarantines, testing, contact tracing, and masking, and its rhetoric ultimately turned much less optimistic. In December 2021, White House COVID-19 Coordinator Jeff Zients warned unvaccinated Americans that they and their families were "looking at a winter of severe illness and death" [21]. By early 2022, many described the Biden administration as having "given up" its pandemic response [22, 23].

What can explain the failure of the world's most powerful nation to contain the spread of COVID-19 and protect its population from exposure and infection? As I suggest in the following discussion, part of the answer lies in influential ideologies regarding American society and Americanness itself. Despite (or perhaps, in part, because of) the humiliations that have accompanied the pandemic, the experience of COVID-19 has seemed to reinvigorate nationalist sentiments in the United States — a trend also observed in other global settings [24]. Yet where nationalism in some regions has reinforced health behaviours — for example, by boosting public pride in the use of face masks [25] — "coronanationalism" in the US has manifested otherwise. Both public and officially led response to the virus has been animated by American exceptionalism — an ideological outlook that one critic describes as an "encompassing state of fantasy" predicated on a belief that the United States is in some way "distinctive", "unique", or "exemplary" [26]. This premise — that the US is the best of the world's nations and stands in a class by itself — has shaped resistance to adopting pandemic control measures that have succeeded elsewhere in the world and underwritten policies that privilege individual liberties at the expense of the collective good. As practiced by actors along the nation's political spectrum, American exceptionalism has proven remarkably corrosive to the implementation of best practices in managing COVID-19.

Public Health as Un-American?

As of June 2022, the time of this writing, the United States has remained a pandemic outlier for the past two and a half years — recording consistently unfavorable epidemiological outcomes under two very different presidential administrations. Through these experiences, one thread has held constant: a disjuncture — or a *perceived* disjuncture — between effective pandemic control and the cultural and political values prized by majoritarian groups in the United States: individualism, self-determination, and freedom from intervention. This sense of cultural misalignment was visible, for example, in the voluble right-wing protests and rallies against masking mandates and stay-at-home orders that were coordinated in many states in 2020.

In the context of the COVID-19 pandemic, advocacy for personal choice, individualism, and freedom from health mandates has been expressed most vocally by right-wing and libertarian groups in the United States, who have seen most public health measures as an infringement on personal sovereignty. The resistance of these groups to pandemic protocols has been positioned as an expression of "medical freedom" — an ideology resting on "an aversion to government interference in personal or family health choices, often coupled to the counter promotion of a spectacular or miracle cure" [27]. Such "therapeutic libertarianism", as Lewis Grossman has called it, has deep historic roots in the US [28]. In the pandemic context, felt sensibilities regarding American civil liberties have underwritten much conservative opposition to the use of face masks. An opinion poll collected in April 2020 suggested that among respondents who chose not to mask, 40% believed it was "their right as an American to not wear a mask" [29]. A later survey of Americans' attitudes towards masking found "protestors believe that mandatory masks are a violation of civil rights" [30].

Owing to the prevalence of anti-masking attitudes among their constituents, Republican governors have tended to rescind state masking orders prematurely, and have often invoked the principles of liberty, freedom, or self-determination when doing so. When Republican governor of Texas Greg Abbott overturned the state's mask mandate in March 2021, he stated that "all businesses and families in Texas have the freedom to determine their own destiny" [31]. The Republican governor of South Dakota made a similar appeal via Twitter: "If folks want to wear a mask, they are free to do so. Those who don't want to wear a mask shouldn't be shamed into it, and govt should not mandate it" [32]. Florida's Republican governor Ron DeSantis similarly framed a 2021 executive order ending mask mandates in public schools as "ensuring parents' freedom to choose." At their most extreme, anti-mask sentiments have further appeared to be arguments for the right to be "anti-hygienic" [33] — or even defenses of "life, liberty, and the pursuit of spitting on other people", in one journalist's phrasing [34]. By their most concerted opponents, face masks have been coded "not as public-minded pandemic reducers, but as speech mufflers" [35].

But more enduringly, if less dramatically, the United States has proven a challenging place to implement any pandemic prevention measures consistently, whether diagnostic testing, contact tracing, quarantine, stay-at-home orders, masking, or vaccination. It is probably fair to say that *no* pandemic mitigation measure has been accepted by Americans without challenge, and some interventions have animated very significant unresolved social and political controversy. Fundamentally, such reticence around COVID-19 measures has rested on an exceptionalist framing of American national identity that valorises the exercise of personal choice — particularly in the form of negative freedoms, or freedoms from outside imposition. Implicitly, this worldview emphasises individualism and — despite its emphasis on the nation as a source of identity and moral orientation — tends to be antagonistic to collectivism.

While right-wing organisations, leaders, and cultural figures have more vocally represented the use of face masks as inimical to traditional American values, preferences, and ways of life, commentators elsewhere on the political spectrum have also contributed to this discourse. Leaders, officials, and public health experts aligned with the Democratic Party have, like their farther-right counterparts, appeared impatient to shed pandemic restrictions — understanding the measures to be unpopular and a potential source of political liability. US government agencies and officials under both presidential administrations, Republican and Democratic, have crafted public health messages that essentially respect anti-masking attitudes. Leaders in both parties have frequently moved to rescind mask mandates prematurely to expedite a return to "business as usual".

Using quieter rhetoric than Republicans, Democratic leaders have also positioned the relaxation of mask measures as a means of restoring a lost Americaness. In an apparent effort to promote unity after the divisive Trump years, President Biden has frequently referenced ideas of shared American identity in his comments on the pandemic and framed individual health behaviours as important to the national interest. Through spring 2021, Biden described masking as a "patriotic duty" and predicted that the roll-out of COVID vaccines would inaugurate a "summer of freedom" to begin on the Fourth of July. Implicitly, the anticipated "freedom" was narrowly defined — more a freedom from masking than the freedom to be healthy as such. But as soon as vaccines for COVID-19 became available to the public [36], Biden largely ceased to comment on masking — despite ongoing calls for "layered protection" in public health — and began emphasising the patriotic nature of vaccination instead. In May 2021, the US Centers for Disease Control (CDC) announced the end of an indoor masking requirement for vaccinated individuals — a move critiqued as premature. Here, Biden explicitly couched the policy shift in terms of both national identity and the nation, stating: "If you're fully vaccinated and can take your mask off, you have earned the right to do something that Americans are known for all around the world: greeting others with a smile. With a smile. So, it is a good day for the country" [37].

While the CDC has vacillated in its recommendations regarding masking, overall its approach has tended — particularly under the Biden administration — to be less protective, and to reframe public health matters in terms of individual concern and personal choice [38]. In early 2022, the United States continued to reach record-breaking levels of morbidity and mortality owing to the ongoing Omicron wave; among the Group of Seven nations, the US ranked first in per-population coronavirus infections and deaths [39]. The national death toll reached 900,000 in the first week of February — yet later that month, the CDC announced a relaxation of indoor masking recommendations on the basis of its newly issued metrics for assessing local COVID risk. The new metrics used hospital capacity — a lagging indicator — instead of treating rates of disease incidence as a key variable defining local risk levels. Many critics understood this both as a concession to the demands of "pandemic minimisers" and an effort to manage appearances in advance of Biden's State of the Union address — an occasion in American political culture that is typically performed with a high level of state pageantry. Despite reports of a new subvariant emerging in Europe and Asia, the President's speech included a curiously triumphalist claim: "Thanks to the progress we have made this past year, COVID-19 need no longer control our lives" [40].

Constructing the "China Virus"

As these events suggest, the use of face masks has remained one of the most contentious concerns surrounding pandemic policy in the US. Though "flu masks" were used by the American public in 1918, the use of face coverings to limit the spread of respiratory illness in daily life is unfamiliar to Americans today [41]. By contrast, everyday masking is commonly found in many East and Southeast Asian countries — particularly since the SARS outbreak in 2003 and the Fukushima nuclear disaster in 2011, but also as protection against more mundane risks like dust, sun, and rhinoviruses. Since 2003 — if not longer — American media have tended to depict the wearing of surgical masks or respirators in everyday settings as foreign and culturally Other. As the co-authors of one study on Japanese masking practices note: "In foreign eyes, mask-wearing appears to be a unique and curious practice particular to Japan. [The] only well-known wearer in the developed world was the late Michael Jackson, identifying the practice with eccentric hypochondria" [42].

Wearing masks has thus been coded as foreign and Asian in mainstream American public perceptions for at least the last two decades. Too, as Hee An Choi and Othelia Lee note, Asian and Asian American populations have long been cast as both "forever foreigners" and sources of disease, as evidenced in the Chinese Exclusion Act of 1882 — a discriminatory federal immigration policy that was not repealed until 1943 [43]. These American perceptual norms — in which face masks are cast as an Asian phenomenon and people of Asian descent are conflated with infectiousness — coincided with media coverage emphasising the Chinese origins of the SARS-CoV-2 virus and characterising the virus as essentially Asian [44]. Over the course of the pandemic, Republican leaders, including senior figures in the Trump administration, have trafficked the epithets "Wuhan virus", "China virus", and "kung flu" [45]. These xenophobic framings were accompanied by a national spike in reported anti-Asian hate crimes [46].

From early moments following the emergence of the novel coronavirus, then, much official commentary has underwritten an ethnocentric and Orientalising account of the pandemic, in which an "ineradicable distinction between Western superiority and Oriental inferiority" is assumed [47]. This worldview was visible in efforts to scapegoat Asian states and settings for the pandemic — including, for example, the widely circulated but never proven theory that SARS-CoV-2 originated from a "lab leak" in Wuhan. In more occulted forms, anti-Asian and Sinophobic views circulated in the mainstream media, avoiding the openly jingoistic, nativistic rhetoric of the Trump administration and its allies. For example, mainstream coverage of a "wet market" in Wuhan, where COVID-19 may have first emerged, tended to recapitulate Orientalist tropes — casting quotidian Asian settings as exotic, unsanitary, and cruel.

Since the third week of March 2020, Asia has outperformed the US, the UK, and the European Union in its rates of cumulative confirmed COVID-19 cases and cumulative confirmed COVID-19 deaths per population [48]. Yet in their coverage of these and other public health achievements by Asian states, Western media have often rested on exceptionalist perspectives — not only casting doubt on reports of positive outcomes, but also positioning Asian strategies of pandemic control as unsuited to Western settings and incompatible with Western values [49]. Throughout, China has been depicted as a potential threat to global health and security — in the form of contagious disease emergence, allegedly misleading official reports, and supposedly incautious scientific agencies — at the same time that it has been cast as a site of irrationally forceful commitments to public health.

In particular, the aspirational "zero-COVID" strategies pursued by multiple Asian states have routinely been criticised in US media — characterised as "impossible" [50] or a "policy nightmare" [51] even when coverage has acknowledged the public health successes these strategies achieved. Few, if any, reports framed experiences in Wuhan, in China, or elsewhere in Asia as a source of policy lessons or tools applicable in the "West". Depicting public response to pandemic control in sensationalising terms — often citing ambient "anger", "anxiety", and "frustration", for example [52] — American journalists and editors have sidestepped the broader rationale informing the zero-COVID approaches that some Asian states have pursued. Casting such policies as repressive political overreach, these accounts equally functioned as a tacit defence of US shortcomings in pandemic control.

Beyond characterising zero-COVID policies as impractical, these reports consistently reinforced an ideological framing of public health measures as restrictive, harsh, unnecessary, and harmful — even violent. For example, Wuhan's lockdown of early 2020 — a political sacrifice that allowed other nations time to prepare — has been consistently positioned in English-language media as "strict", "severe", "aggressive", "authoritarian", "brutal", and even "dictatorial"; not as a necessary evil or a gift to the international community, and still less as an important precedent in controlling COVID-19 [53–55]. Much of this coverage has tacitly drawn on mainstream American stereotypes of Asians as "competent but not warm" [56], depicting Chinese authorities as technocratic, impersonal, and inhumane. For example, in December 2021, a *Washington Post* report characterised a lockdown in the city of Xi'an as "severe", even as it reported the government's coordination of food deliveries [57]. Along similar lines, a *Reuters* journalist characterised the 2022 Winter Olympics in Beijing as "dystopian", disparagingly citing attendee policies intended to minimise the risk of COVID exposure and transmission [58]. One policy analyst argued: "No other nation (…) can or should seek to replicate China's actions", suggesting that the lockdowns were of a piece with the outbreak's very origins [59].

As these experiences suggest, US leaders, media, and part of the American public have attempted to manage the COVID-19 pandemic via rhetoric that is essentially neo-Orientalist — depicting Asian nations as politically and culturally alien and derogating the efforts of China, in particular, to respond to the pandemic within its own borders. At the same time, American journalists, policy commentators, and leaders have discursively constructed the United States and its culture of civic freedoms in exceptionalising contradistinction to an imaginary of East Asia that is characterised as both socially primitive and tyrannically modern.

Conclusion: An Encompassing State of Fantasy?

Over the past two and a half years and under two presidential administrations, COVID-19 response in the US has deviated significantly from the gold standard of pandemic response capacity that assessments like the GHSI presumed. While some of these lapses may be attributed to populist leadership under the Trump administration in 2020, many early missteps in the nation's pandemic response — as well as counterproductive trends in popular opinion, public health behaviours, and media reporting — have continued under the Biden administration.

Despite making fewer egregious missteps, currently US pandemic response continues to be shaped by libertarian ideals, a narrowly defined version of individual freedoms, and a felt sense of ethnic and national superiority vis-à-vis East Asia and other world regions. Yet the country's deeply troubled pandemic response and high levels of morbidity and mortality have barely appeared to dent the "encompassing state of fantasy" of American pandemic exceptionalism. Absent a concerted effort to address the roots of these failures, it seems probable that the nation will continue recording public health outcomes far inferior to those achieved elsewhere — while continuing to promote a US-centric vision that makes a virtue of uniquely American shortcomings.

References

[1] Andrew, S (2020, June 30). The US has 4% of the world's population but 25% of its coronavirus cases. *CNN*. https://www.cnn.com/2020/06/30/health/us-coronavirus-toll-in-numbers-june-trnd/index.html.

[2] Gostin, L & Wetter, S (2020, March 31). Why there's no national lockdown. *The Atlantic*. https://www.theatlantic.com/ideas/archive/2020/03/why-theres-no-national-lockdown/609127/.

[3] Tracking covid-19 across the world (2021, April 21). *The Economist*. https://www.economist.com/graphic-detail/tracking-coronavirus-across-the-world.

[4] Trends in number of COVID-19 vaccinations in the US (2022, June 14). *Centers for Disease Control*. https://covid.cdc.gov/covid-data-tracker/#vaccination-trends_vacctrends-fully-daily.

[5] Mandavilli, A (2022, April 26). The coronavirus has infected more than half of Americans, the C.D.C. reports. *New York Times*. https://www.nytimes.com/2022/04/26/health/coronavirus-antibodies-americans-cdc.html.

[6] While establishing that no country appeared perfectly prepared to contend with a novel pathogen, the GHSI ranking system rated the United States highly across six domains and assigned the US an overall score of 83.5 out of 100 — ranking it ahead of the United Kingdom, the Netherlands, Australia, Canada, Thailand, and Sweden [60].

[7] Elliott, L (2020, April 22). Top economist: US coronavirus response is like 'third world' country. *The Guardian*. https://www.theguardian.com/business/2020/apr/22/top-economist-us-coronavirus-response-like-third-world-country-joseph-stiglitz-donald-trump.

[8] Mortality analyses (2022). *Johns Hopkins University Coronavirus Resource Center*. https://coronavirus.jhu.edu/data/mortality.

[9] Mueller, B & Lutz, E (2022, February 1). U.S. has far higher Covid death rate than other wealthy countries. *New York Times*. https://www.nytimes.com/interactive/2022/02/01/science/covid-deaths-united-states.html.

[10] Bilinski, A & Emanuel, EJ (2022). COVID-19 and excess all-cause mortality in the US and 18 comparison countries. *JAMA*, **324**(20), 2100–2102.

[11] Maxmen, A & Tollefson, J (2020, August 4). Two decades of pandemic war games failed to account for Donald Trump. *Nature*. https://www.nature.com/articles/d41586-020-02277-6.

[12] Noel, TK (2020). Conflating culture with COVID-19: Xenophobic repercussions of a global pandemic. *Social Sciences & Humanities*, **2**(1), 100044.

[13] Schaefer, BJ (2021). "I don't think the science knows, actually": The biocultural impacts of Trump's anti-science and misinformation rhetoric, the mishandling of the COVID-19 pandemic, and institutionalized racism. In Eller, JD (Ed.), *The Anthropology of Donald Trump: Culture and the Exceptional Moment*, pp. 161–181. Routledge.

[14] Miller, Z (2020, September 9). 'Deadly stuff': Trump's own words bring focus back to virus. *AP News*. https://apnews.com/article/pandemics-donald-trump-bob-woodward-elections-virus-outbreak-cb579c89907b73e546459848e2b3bb67.

[15] The United States was not the only nation whose head of state advanced anti-science sentiments. As medical anthropologist Gideon Lasco has argued, Trump — like his illiberal counterparts in Brazil and the Philippines — conveyed messages of "medical populism" in response to COVID: "simplifying the pandemic by downplaying its impacts or touting easy solutions or treatments, spectacularizing their responses to crisis, forging divisions between the 'people' and dangerous 'others,' and making medical knowledge claims to support the above" [16].

[16] Lasco, G (2020). Medical populism and the COVID-19 pandemic. *Global Public Health*, **15**(10), 1417-1429.

[17] Leonhardt, D & Leatherby, L (2020, June 2). Where the virus is growing most: Countries with 'illiberal populist' leaders. *New York Times*. https://www.nytimes.com/2020/06/02/briefing/coronavirus-populist-leaders.html.

[18] Cepaluni, G, Dorsch, MT, & Branyiczki, R (2022). Political regimes and deaths in the early stages of the COVID-19 pandemic. *Journal of Public Finance and Public Choice*, **37**(1), 27–53.

[19] Hamblin, J (2022, March 12). Can public health be saved? *New York Times*. https://www.nytimes.com/2022/03/12/opinion/public-health-trust.html.

[20] Knight, V & Appleby, J (2021, September 15). Biden releases a new plan to combat Covid, but experts say there's still a ways to go. *KHN*. https://khn.org/news/article/biden-promise-tracker-vaccination-progress-plan-to-get-covid-under-control/.

[21] Press briefing by White House COVID-19 response team and public health officials (2021, December 17). *White House*. https://www.whitehouse.gov/briefing-room/press-briefings/2021/12/17/press-briefing-by-white-house-covid-19-response-team-and-public-health-officials-74/.

[22] Gonsalves, G (2022, March 10). The Biden administration turns its back on the pandemic. *The Nation*. https://www.thenation.com/article/society/covid-biden-policy-abdandonment/.

[23] Wu, K (2022, March 2). The Biden administration killed America's collective pandemic approach. *The Atlantic*. https://www.theatlantic.com/health/archive/2022/03/covid-cdc-guidelines-masks/623337/.

[24] Gustavsson, G (2020, May 3). The risk of Sweden's coronavirus strategy? Blind patriotism. *Washington Post*. https://www.washingtonpost.com/politics/2020/05/03/risk-swedens-coronavirus-strategy-blind-patriotism/.

[25] Goode, J, Stroup, D & Gaufman, E (2022). Everyday nationalism in unsettled times: In search of normality during pandemic. *Nationalities Papers*, **50**(1), 61–85.

[26] Pease, D (2009). *The New American Exceptionalism*. University of Minnesota Press.

[27] Hotez, P (2021). America's deadly flirtation with antiscience and the medical freedom movement. *The Journal of Clinical Investigation*, **131**(7), e149072.

[28] Grossman, LA (2013). The origins of American health libertarianism. *Yale Journal of Health Policy, Law, and Ethics*, **13**(1), 76–134.

[29] American individualism is an obstacle to wider mask wearing in the US (2020, August 31). *Brookings Institution*. https://www.brookings.edu/blog/up-front/2020/08/31/american-individualism-is-an-obstacle-to-wider-mask-wearing-in-the-us/.

[30] Taylor, S & Amundson, G (2021). Negative attitudes about facemasks during the COVID-19 pandemic: The dual importance of perceived ineffectiveness and psychological reactance. *PloS One*, **16**(2), e0246317.

[31] Governor Abbott lifts mask mandate, opens Texas 100 percent (2021, March 2). *Office of the Texas Governor*. https://gov.texas.gov/news/post/governor-abbott-lifts-mask-mandate-opens-texas-100-percent.

[32] Hotez, P (2021, January 28). Anti-science kills: From Soviet embrace of pseudoscience to accelerated attacks on US biomedicine. *PLoS Biology*, **19**(1), e3001068.

[33] Vieten, U (2020). The "new normal" and "pandemic populism": The COVID-19 crisis and anti-hygienic mobilisation of the far-right. *Social Science*, **9**(9), 165.

[34] Gessen, M (2020, May 26). Life, liberty, and the pursuit of spitting on other people. *The New Yorker*. https://www.newyorker.com/news/our-columnists/life-liberty-and-the-pursuit-of-spitting-on-other-people/amp.

[35] Bratich, J (2021). 'Give me liberty or give me Covid!': Antilockdown protests as necropopulist downsurgency. *Cultural Studies*, **35**(2–3), 257–265.

[36] Remarks by President Biden on the fight against COVID-19 (2021, December 21). *White House*. https://www.whitehouse.gov/briefing-room/speeches-remarks/2021/12/21/remarks-by-president-biden-on-the-fight-against-covid-19/.

[37] Gittleson, B and Gomez, J (2021). 'A great day for America,' Biden says, touting CDC's eased mask guidance. *ABC News*. https://abcnews.go.com/Politics/great-day-america-biden-touting-cdcs-eased-mask/story?id=77673806.

[38] Tomori, C, et al. (2021). Your health is in your hands? US CDC COVID-19 mask guidance reveals the moral foundations of public health. *eClinicalMedicine*, **38**, 101071.

[39] Schreiber, M (2022, February 6). Vastly unequal U.S. has world's highest COVID death toll — It's no coincidence. *The Guardian*. https://www.theguardian.com/us-news/2022/feb/06/us-covid-death-rate-vaccines.

[40] State of the Union Address (2022, March 1). *White House*. https://www.whitehouse.gov/state-of-the-union-2022/.

[41] The first surgical masks were designed and put into use in late 19th-century Europe [61], but the first use of masks by the general public took place during a pneumonic plague

outbreak in Manchuria in 1910 [62]. In 1918, responding to the H1N1 flu pandemic, some American municipalities mandated masking — but mask use has not been practiced among the general public since, even during the 2009 influenza A (H1N1) pandemic [63].

[42] Burgess, A & Horii, M (2012). Risk, ritual and health responsibilisation: Japan's 'safety blanket' of surgical face mask-wearing. *Sociology of Health & Illness*, **34**(8), 1184–1198.

[43] Choi, HA & Lee, OE (2021). To mask or to unmask, that is the question: Facemasks and anti-Asian violence during COVID-19. *Journal of Human Rights and Social Work*, **6**, 237–245.

[44] These representations closely paralleled Western media coverage of the SARS outbreak in 2003, which also trafficked in othering and exceptionalising rhetoric and portrayed "China and the Chinese as an inevitable breeding ground for new infections" [64].

[45] Haiphong, D (2020). The great unmasking: American exceptionalism in the age of COVID-19. *International Critical Thought*, **10**(2), 200–213.

[46] Gover, AR, Harper, SB & Langton, L (2020). Anti-Asian hate crime during the COVID-19 pandemic: Exploring the reproduction of inequality. *American Journal of Criminal Justice*, **45**, 647–667.

[47] Said, E (1978). *Orientalism*. Pantheon Books.

[48] *COVID-19 Data Explorer* (2022). *Our World in Data*. https://ourworldindata.org/coronavirus.

[49] Leung, H (2020, March 20). Why wearing a face mask is encouraged in Asia, but shunned in the U.S. *TIME*. https://time.com/5799964/coronavirus-face-mask-asia-us/.

[50] Frost, R, Zhao, S & Curran, E (2022, February 10). Hong Kong risks everything with 'impossible' Covid-Zero goal. *Bloomberg Businessweek*. https://www.bloomberg.com/news/articles/2022-02-10/hong-kong-is-risking-everything-with-zealous-covid-zero-pursuit.

[51] Lau, J (2022, February 18). The end game of China's zero-COVID policy nightmare. *WIRED*. https://www.wired.com/story/china-zero-covid-vaccines/.

[52] Chang, A, Qin, A, Qian, I & Chien, AC (2022, April 29). Under lockdown in China. *New York Times*. https://www.nytimes.com/interactive/2022/04/29/world/asia/shanghai-lockdown.html.

[53] Gostin, L & Wetter, S (2020, March 31). Why there's no national lockdown. *The Atlantic*. https://www.theatlantic.com/ideas/archive/2020/03/why-theres-no-national-lockdown/609127/.

[54] Mozur, P (2020, February 3). China, desperate to stop coronavirus, turns neighbor against neighbor. *New York Times*. https://www.nytimes.com/2020/02/03/business/china-coronavirus-wuhan-surveillance.html.

[55] Kupferschmidt, K & Cohen, J (2020, March 2). China's aggressive measures have slowed the coronavirus. They may not work in other countries. *Science*. https://www.science.org/content/article/china-s-aggressive-measures-have-slowed-coronavirus-they-may-not-work-other-countries.

[56] Cuddy, AJC, Fiske, ST & Glick, P (2007). The BIAS map: Behaviors from intergroup affect and stereotypes. *Journal of Personality and Social Psychology*, **92**(4), 631–648.

[57] Dou, E (2021, December 21). Locked down in China's Xi'an amid coronavirus outbreak, residents subsist on deliveries of vegetables. *Washington Post*. https://www. washingtonpost.com/world/2021/12/30/china-covid-lockdown-xian/.

[58] Saito, M [@saitomri] (2022, February 3). Hello, I wrote about the EXTREMELY dystopian vibes inside the bubble at the Beijing Olympics. Exhibit A: Hotel bartenders making [Tweet]. *Twitter*. https://twitter.com/saitomri/status/1489151047507800064?s=20&t=0B lylHVSUyHlhj4BcwvL2w.

[59] Gunia, A (2020, March 13). China's draconian lockdown is getting credit for slowing coronavirus. Would it work anywhere else? *TIME*. https://time.com/5796425/china-coronavirus-lockdown/.

[60] Global Health Security Index: Building collective action and accountability (2019). *Nuclear Threat Initiative*. https://www.ghsindex.org/wp-content/uploads/2019/10/2019-Global-Health-Security-Index.pdf.

[61] Hare, R (1964). The transmission of respiratory diseases. *Royal Society of Medicine*, **57**(3), 222.

[62] Lynteris, C (2018). Plague masks: The visual emergence of anti-epidemic personal protection equipment, *Medical Anthropology*, **37**(6), 442–457.

[63] Parker-Pope, T (2009, May 4). Worry? Relax? Buy face mask? Answers on flu. *New York Times*. https://www.nytimes.com/2009/05/05/health/05well.html.

[64] Washer, P (2004). Representations of SARS in the British newspapers. *Social Science and Medicine*, 59(12), 2561–2571.

Chapter

6

What Do Four Waves of COVID Tell Us?

By David Meenagh and Patrick Minford

Summary

Using the unique, recently made public sample-based estimates of infections produced by the Office for National Statistics (ONS), this research extends Meenagh and Minford [1] to the four waves of illness in the UK by the end of 2021. These allow us to estimate the effects on the COVID hospitalisation and fatality rates of vaccination and population immunity due to past infection: the latter was the most significant factor driving both trends, while the vaccination rate also had a significant short-run effect on the fatality rate. For the most recent data, we again updated our policy comparison with Sweden and came to the same conclusions: in waves 1 and 2, reduced Swedish lockdown intensity compared to personal response resulted in much lower economic costs with no appreciable impact on infections.

Introduction

In two earlier studies [1, 2] we presented a structural model to describe how the COVID virus would spread in the UK and Sweden using optimised households, biologically optimised virus behaviour, and pertinent governmental actions. Since the UK's more interventionist approach led to different outcomes for infections and mortality, we focused on how Sweden's policy framework, which was fundamentally different, differed from the UK's.

82

In our first paper, we analysed data on the first wave of infection in both nations; in our second paper, we expanded this analysis to include the three or four waves through the end of 2021. In this chapter, we provide a non-technical summary of this research, examine its findings, and identify its most important policy recommendations.

According to evolutionary biology, respiratory viruses evolve to become more contagious and less harmful to health, implying a lower fatality rate because both of these changes should boost their chances of surviving. If this is the case, we should observe the rate of transmission increasing over the course of the four waves with the death rate per case decreasing, both independently of the advancements in vaccination, which were rolled out quickly in the UK before and during the third wave and slightly more slowly in Sweden. Indeed, from case data, we already know that the transmissibility increased with each new variant. For example, in the UK's second wave, this evidence showed that the "Kent variant", which predominated, was 50% more transmissible than the original (first wave) virus, and that the D-variant, which predominated in the third wave, was again 50–60% more transmissible than the Kent variant. Evidence about the UK fatality rate has been more difficult to locate, in part because the amount of testing has had an impact on the case numbers as estimated by the National Health Service (NHS). In our most recent work, we used ONS estimates of infections, which are based on a fixed sampling basis rather than on people who take tests. We then combined these from their starting point in May 2020 with the NHS data prior to that, together with data from the website ZOE (see www.joinzoe.com) on self-reported symptoms, in order to create a complete data set across all four UK waves. This preliminary data should be devoid of test bias since it records illnesses rather than test takers. Since we do not have sample-based data for Sweden and only have access to Johns Hopkins data from reported cases that are obtained from Swedish health sources, we created an infection series from the death data using UK estimates of the infection fatality rate for the variant of the time to find implied infections. Thus, for the estimation of structural and reduced form models over the whole COVID history for both the UK and Sweden, we have used a complete and relatively accurate collection of data in this study; our goal has been to develop more accurate predictions of these virus characteristics as well as the results of other interventions like immunisation. We derive new policy conclusions from this updated set of estimates.

The Model — A Non-Technical Account

You can find a detailed technical description of the model in [1]. Here, we provide a non-mathematical explanation of how it functions. The virus, whose evolutionary nature is thought to maximise its chances of survival, is one of the two key agents in the model. The population's fundamental resilience to infection (γ) and governmental actions like lockdown that prevent infection (μ) are the major parameters fighting against this. Additionally, the virus encounters household evasion strategies, or ξ_t, as optimised by households in their own virus-fighting tactics. Vaccination also directly enters the model through the parameter χ by preventing infection.

The household behaviour in the model assumes that household utility is reduced by infection but also by the personal inconvenience of avoiding infection by self-isolation activity, ξ_t. As this increases, the individual costs of not participating in social and economic activities rise directly with the degree of isolation and indirectly with the number of uninfected individuals because participation reduces the individual risk of infection, which raises the net costs of self-isolation (the economic costs net of the gain in lower infection risk). The parameter ϕ determines how these net costs respond to the accumulation of infected individuals; as it rises, they react to increased infection more forcefully, indicating that they isolate themselves more actively as infection levels rise. Households maximise this utility with respect to ξ_t subject to the virus's behaviour set out above, so they take account of the virus's behaviour.

Data and Results for UK

The indirect inference method is used to estimate and test the model (see [3] for more details). Similar to the simulated method of moments, this method is simulation-based. In order to evaluate the model, we first utilise an 'auxiliary model' whose role is to describe the data, and we then determine how closely the auxiliary model's parameters derived from the real data agree with those calculated from the simulated model as a whole. The model is not rejected and is a reasonable descriptor of the data if the actual data coefficients fall within the 95% bounds of the distribution of coefficients from the simulated data. During estimation the structural model parameters are varied until a set is found with the highest p-value. This set of parameters would be the closest to the data. In this study, the auxiliary model is a logistic function with the following form, fitted to infections:

$$f(x,a,b,c) = \frac{c}{1+e^{-(x-b)/a}}$$

where x is time, and the three parameters are:

a is the infection speed;

b is the day when the maximum number of new infections occurred;

c is the total number of recorded infected people at the end of the infections.

These are the three parameters we try to match in the Indirect Inference procedure.

Table 6.1 shows the estimated structural parameters for the three waves under consideration.

We observe that the parameters of Waves 1 and 2 are remarkably similar. The lockdown factor, μ, is a significant multiple of the personal reaction factor, ϕ, in both cases, showing significant lockdown interventions. The estimations drastically alter with the third and fourth waves as a result of the vaccination roll-out. Because so many people are immunised, the level of immunity, γ, increases dramatically. μ also increases because the virus's resistance rises with higher penetration. Additionally, ϕ rises, because the vaccine has given individuals more confidence, so they are responding much more favourably to increased penetration. Naturally, the spread of the vaccination itself has an impact on the virus's development that was not present in earlier waves.

Table 6.1 Structural model parameter estimates for the three waves.

	Wave 1	Wave 2	Waves 3–4
γ	74.8847	68.9229	85.5612
μ	3.3705	3.594	5.3381
a	−9.3384	−5.1107	−8.4966
ϕ	0.1457	0.3192	0.927
μ/ϕ	23.1	11.3	5.8
χ	NA	0.1947	0.761
$(\mu + \phi)/(\gamma + \phi)$	0.047	0.056	0.071
p-value	0.9639	0.0827	0.0574

Table 6.2   Results for total infected (millions).

	Actual c	Model Mean c	Model Steady-State	Data
Wave 1	4.5	6.6	4.7	4.7
Wave 2	18.6	16.1	18.2	18.2
Wave 3	19.8	14.4	17.3	17.3

The three waves differ in the overall numbers infected (see Table 6.4 below for exact dates of each wave):

In Table 6.2, we can see that the model mean roughly matches the logistic c value, and the steady state of the model is bound in estimation (by the constant) to equal the sum of the data. It is remarkable how few people were infected during the first wave compared to the following two, where approximately four and a half times as many people were.

However, the number of deaths in the first two waves was roughly similar, highlighting how high the initial death rate was and how much it decreased in the second wave (by a factor of 4). Figure 6.1 illustrates how the death rate decreased steadily throughout all waves, reaching a significantly reduced rate by the third wave after immunisation.

Analysing Trends in the Hospitalisation and Death Rates of the UK

Figure 6.2 shows the evolution of two ratios: deaths to hospitalisations and hospitalisations to infections, where hospitalisations are measured by those in hospital. The bottom plot in Figure 6.2 displays the projected COVID prevalence. As we move through the waves, the ratios appear to be declining even while the projected number of infected is rising. The vertical lines show the end of each wave and the start of the next.

How the hospitalisation and death rates will change is the crucial question as Wave 4 progresses. It is possible to keep "living with COVID" if these are disconnected from the infection rate. However, if they continue to be high enough to cause an excessive amount of hospital admissions and fatalities, additional lockdown interventions will be compelled to return to the agenda.

We investigate this by regressing hospitalisation/cases on the double-vaccination rate, the cumulative infection rate as a proportion of the population

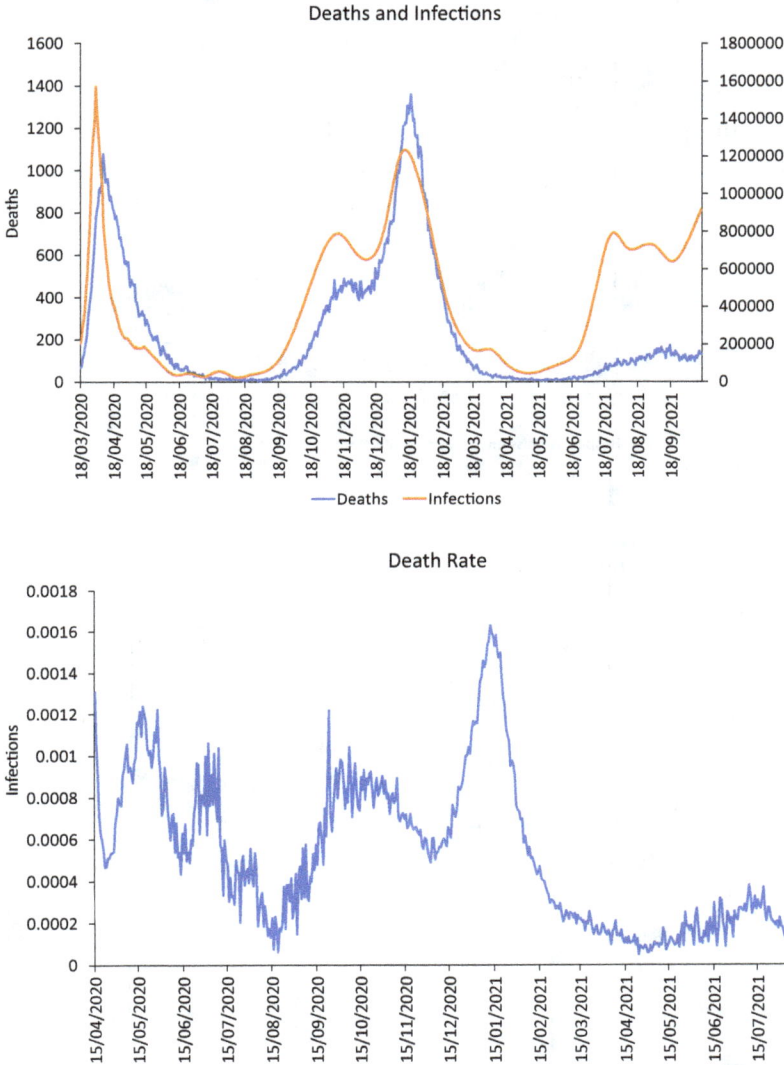

Figure 6.1 Deaths and infections.

(PCINF, to proxy growing immunity), and the population's overall vaccination rate (VACC, a weighted average of the percentage of the population who have had either two or three vaccinations). Then we repeat the process for deaths/ lagged hospitalisations; here, PCINF will also capture the impact of new treatments that have developed as a result of infection experience. We might also see a result of the higher booster rate for Wave 4 numbers.

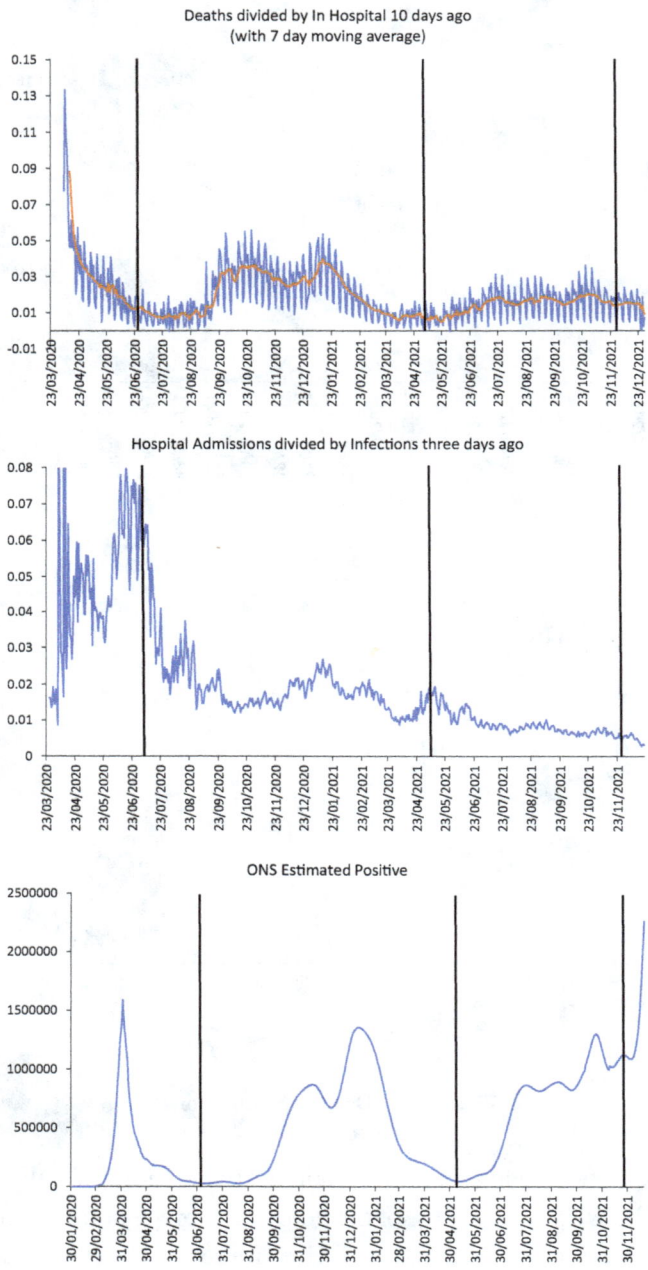

Figure 6.2   Data on infections, hospitalisation and deaths over the four waves.

Figure 6.3 shows the percentage of the population that have COVID and the percentage of the population that are vaccinated.

We used extensive UK data on estimated cases, hospitalisations, and deaths to regress the hospitalisation ratio to lagged infections and the deaths ratio to lagged hospitalisations to understand the potential influences of vaccines and immunity on the changing statistics. Although immunity should have an

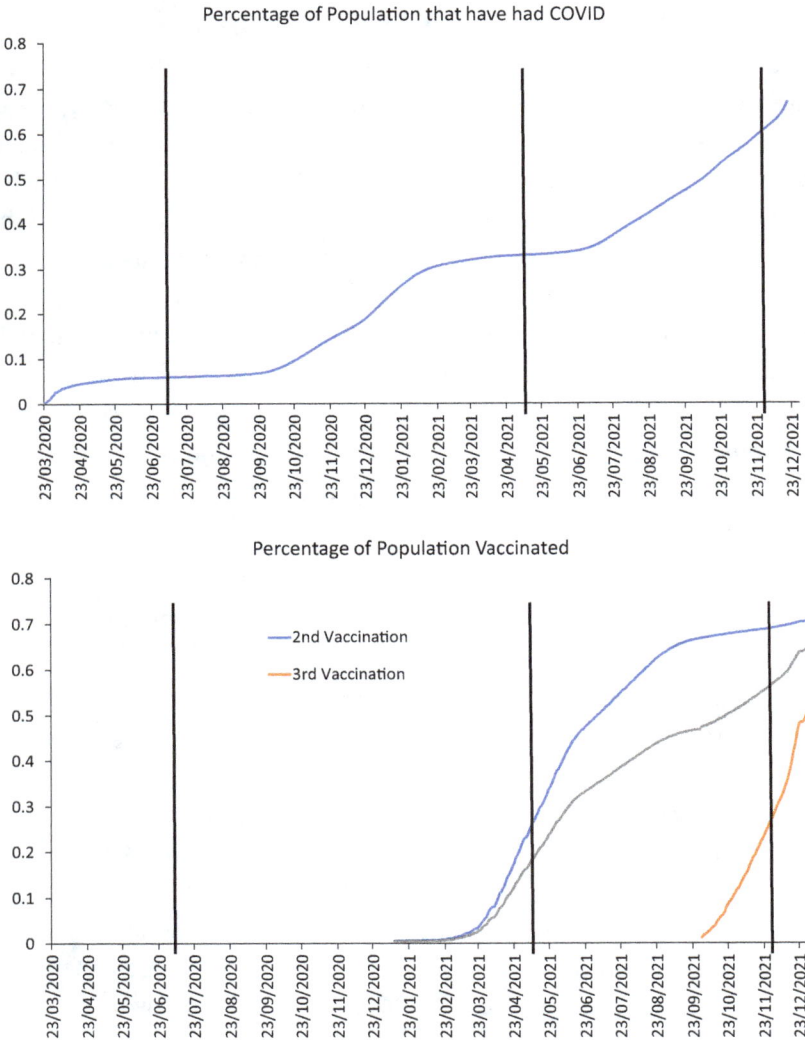

Figure 6.3   Vaccinations and infections.

increasing impact as the virus gets older, we would anticipate that vaccinations would have a consistent impact. We estimate — Table 6.3 — both long-run relationships ('cointegrating' equations where the level of the dependent variable is regressed on the levels of the exogenous variables) and short-run ones (the Error-Correcting Model where changes in the dependent variable are regressed on changes in the exogenous ones and also on past deviations of the dependent variable from its long-run relationship).

We discovered that the vaccination rate and the overall previous total infection rate, which serve as proxies for the developed immunity, have cointegrating relationships to both the hospitalisation (*i.e.*, those in the hospital) ratio to infections and the mortality ratio to hospitalisations. Additionally, we discover an error-correcting equation that clearly links the change in these series to the recent vaccine shocks (which are negative), recent infections (which are positive), and the lagged deviation from trend (which is negative); all of these effects are substantial. When the various vaccine components are weighted together to create a meaningful vaccine variable, these regressions suggest that vaccinations, however, were less significant than immunity (proxied by the cumulative total/population of those infected, PCINF) in reducing the trends in hospital/cases and in deaths/those in hospital. In both cointegrating regressions, the VACC weighted variable is not significant, although PCINF is significant and correctly signed in both. The early tendency of hospitalisation

Table 6.3   Trends in the virus behaviour.

	IHI3	DIH10
Long-Run Relationship		
Constant	0.387331***	0.025383***
VACC	−0.048440	0.002388
PCINF	−0.639231***	−0.023662***
ECM Regression		
Constant	0.017141	−0.002265***
Δ(VACC)	−3.59375	−0.717900***
Δ(PCINF)	−13.1755	2.803055***
Long Run Residual(−1)	−0.482439***	−0.393575***
Cointegrating ADF p-value	0.003666	0.023863

IHI3 = (In Hospital)/Infections(−3), DIH10 = Deaths/(In Hospital(−10))
***$p < 0.01$, **$p < 0.05$, *$p < 0.10$

and death rates to decline well before vaccination started is being picked up by this trend effect in PCINF. However, both variables also have substantial short-term effects. Therefore, both have a crucial role. These regressions imply that immunity played a greater role in reversing the trends in hospital admissions and mortality than vaccinations did. In both cointegrating regressions, the VACC weighted variable is not significant, although PCINF is significant and correctly signed in both.

Data and Results for Sweden

The number of reported cases from the Swedish Health Agency and deaths reported via Johns Hopkins are shown in Figure 6.4. For Sweden, Wave 1

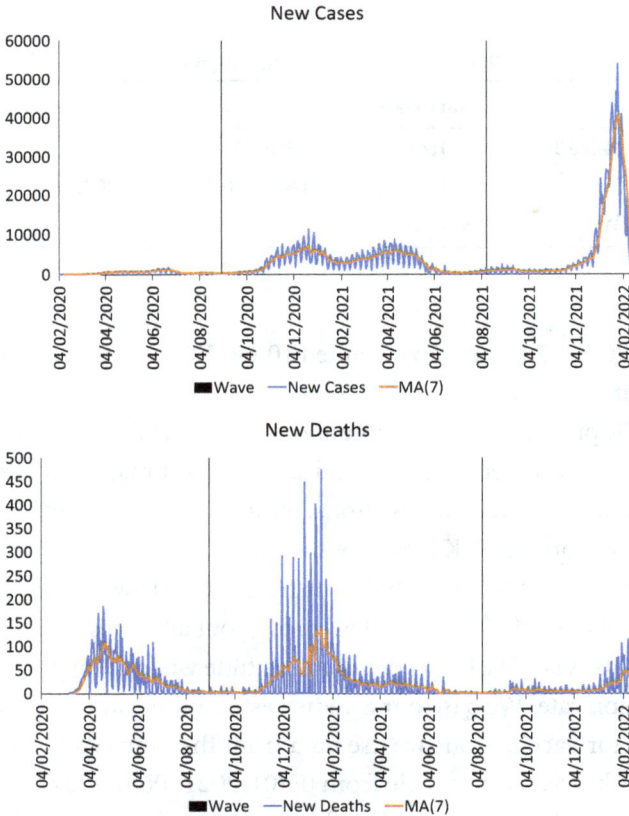

Figure 6.4 Swedish COVID cases and deaths.

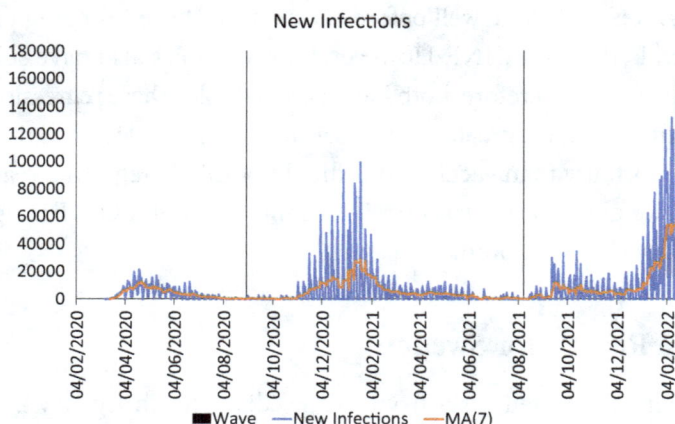

Figure 6.5   Estimated Swedish COVID infections.

Table 6.4   Death rate for UK waves.

	Start Date	End Date	Death Rate
Wave 1	30/01/2020	05/07/2020	0.008542
Wave 2	06/07/2020	08/05/2021	0.004769
Wave 3	09/05/2021		0.000863

ended on 01/09/2020, and Wave 2 ended 10/08/2021, as shown by the vertical lines in Figures 6.4 and 6.5.

Given the probable mortality rate and the data on fatalities, it would appear that the Swedish cases represent a significant underestimation of infections. So, in order to estimate Swedish infections, we use UK death rates. Total deaths/ total infections for each UK wave are shown in Table 6.4.

If we apply these to Swedish deaths from COVID we obtain Figure 6.5.

With a total of 5,126,659 infected throughout all waves—roughly half the population—this is a feasible order of magnitude when compared to the UK's ~65% infection rate. We base our Swedish estimations on this infection data.

Finally, for vaccinations we use data from the Our World in Data database [4]. Weekly data is available from 03/01/2021–06/02/2022, and the data available at irregular frequency after this date, therefore we have interpolated the data to a daily frequency (Figure 6.6).

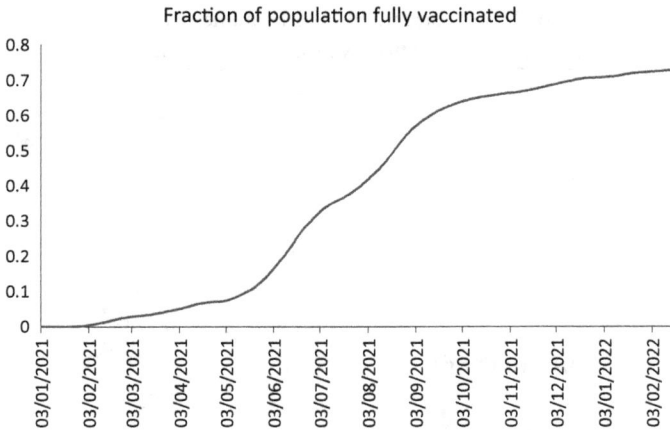

Figure 6.6 Fraction of Swedish population fully vaccinated.

Estimates of Swedish Model

After estimating the model for the four waves, we found that the model could not fit for Waves 3 and 4. This might be due to the fact that the data for these waves do not resemble an S-shaped logistic function; rather, they more closely resemble the beginning of an incomplete wave. As a result, they do not suit our auxiliary model, which is applicable to an entirely finished wave. Table 6.5 displays the structural parameters. With a p-value of 0.458 for Wave 1, we discovered that the model matches the data very well. With a p-value of 0.1554, the models also fit Wave 2 well, however it slightly overpredicts the auxiliary model's c coefficient.

In our previous estimates shown in [1] for Sweden, which were based on deaths and were directly comparable with our UK estimates also based on deaths, we found that the lockdown parameter for the UK was much larger than Sweden's, while the personal response parameter was much smaller. Thus the ratio of the lockdown to the personal response parameter, which summarises the policy contrast, was much lower in Sweden than in the UK — at 0.05 *vs* 24.2, respectively. According to our most recent estimates for Sweden, shown in Table 6.5, the comparison with the UK based on our less comparable estimates from the new data no longer holds on average across the first two waves for the absolute values of the lockdown parameter and does with less

Table 6.5   Structural model parameter estimates for the first two waves for Sweden.

	Wave 1	Wave 2
γ	149.0657	138.8889
μ	6.3528	1.437
α	−19.1283	−2.2917
ϕ	0.7525	0.2541
μ/ϕ	8.44	5.65
χ	NA	0.1445
$(\mu + \phi)/(\gamma + \phi)$	0.047	0.011
Wald	2.3474	5.232
p-value	0.458	0.1554

pronounced contrast for the absolute values of the personal one; but for the ratio it continues to show fairly substantial contrast, averaging around 7 for Sweden as opposed to 17 for the UK. The Swedish ratio also resembles that for wave 3/4 in the UK (at 5.6), which corresponds with the UK's policy change from lockdown to vaccination. Therefore, the most recent findings are broadly consistent with our earlier ones and with what we know about the policies of the two countries on the key policy question of the use of mandated *vs* advisory intervention.

Economic Costs of COVID Policies

In our first study, we noted that Sweden's COVID policies, based on less direct intervention and more advice for personal behaviour, resulted in significantly lower first-wave economic costs while essentially maintaining the infection's course. With our new estimates, we discover the same thing here. Figure 6.7 illustrates how Sweden's less interventionist strategy in Waves 1 and 2 led to a substantially smaller GDP decline in comparison to its pre-COVID level. The UK's approach abandoned lockdown in favour of vaccination and advice in waves 3/4, to conform to Sweden's.

Again, the updated pattern of the two countries' cumulative infections is hard to distinguish, as Figure 6.8 shows.

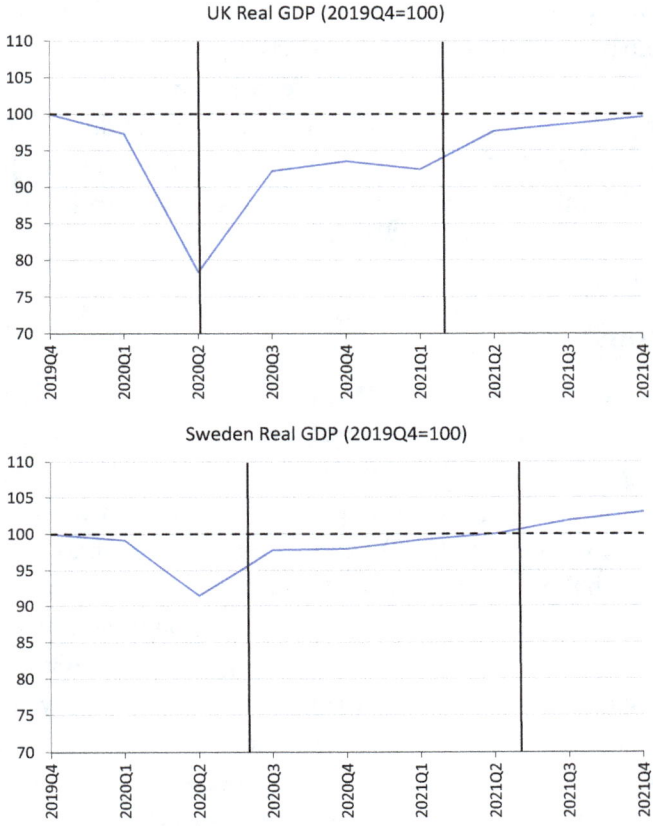

Figure 6.7   Real GDP during the COVID waves.

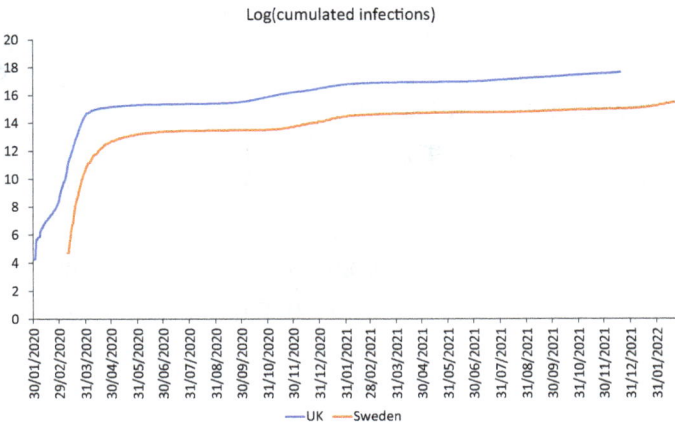

Figure 6.8   Cumulative infections (in log) for UK and Sweden.

What we observe is that on average, during Wave 1, UK GDP decreased by 8.5% from pre-COVID (2019 Q4) levels, compared to a decrease of 3.8% for Swedish GDP; during Wave 2, UK GDP decreased by 8.5% from pre-COVID levels, compared to a decrease of 1.1% for Sweden; and during Wave 3, UK GDP decreased by 1.7% , compared to a rise of 2.2% for Sweden. The average loss from UK policy compared to Sweden's was 5.3% for the course of the pandemic as a whole, considering each wave equally.

Conclusions

In this research using the COVID transmission model presented earlier [1, 2], we have extended our empirical estimates to the whole data on the pandemic up to the end of 2021, by which time there had been four waves of infection in the UK. In place of the previously utilised infections estimated from fatalities, we used the ONS's recently made sample-based estimates of infections. With the aid of these updated and trustworthy estimates, we were also able to link vaccinations and acquired population immunity from earlier infections to the disease's progression, including the hospitalisation and fatality rates. Finally, in order to reflect the most recent statistics, we revised our comparison with Sweden. Unfortunately, there are no comparable sample-based data for infections — as far as we are aware, the ONS sample survey approach has not been used anywhere else in the world.

Our most recent findings remain largely consistent with those of our earlier studies: in the first two waves, the Swedish lockdown's intensity in terms of personal response was significantly lower than that of the UK, resulting in significantly lower economic costs while making little difference to the disease's course. By wave 3/4, the UK had left lockdown, which caused its projected relative intensity to decline along with it and decrease economic costs.

We discovered that the population's accumulated infection rate, a gauge of its herd immunity, was the most significant factor influencing trends in hospitalisation and fatalities based on our distinctive UK sample-based data. The fatality rate was significantly impacted in the short term by the vaccination rate as well.

References

[1] Meenagh, D & Minford, P (2021). A structural model of coronavirus behaviour for testing on data behaviour. *Applied Economics*, **53**(30), 3515–3534.

[2] Meenagh, D & Minford, P (2022). A structural model of coronavirus behaviour for testing on data behaviour — what do four waves of data tell us?. *Applied Economics*, in press. https://doi.org/10.1080/00036846.2022.2128295.

[3] Le, VPM, Meenagh, D, Minford, P, Wickens, M & Xu, Y (2016). Testing macro models by indirect inference: a survey for users. *Open Economies Review*, **27**(1), 1–38.

[4] Mathieu, E, Ritchie, H, Ortiz-Ospina, E, Roser, M, Hasell, J, Appel, C, Giattino, C & Rodés-Guirao, L (2021). A global database of COVID-19 vaccinations. *Nature Human Behaviour*, **5**, 947–953.

https://doi.org/10.1142/9789811262821_0007

Chapter

7

Trust the Public? How the UK Government Got the Psychology of COVID-19 Wrong and Why It Matters

By Stephen Reicher

Summary

In this chapter I examine the role of trust in the response of the UK Government to the COVID-19 pandemic. I start by showing the importance of trust to a successful response. I then document the Government's lack of trust in the reactions of the public, which was rooted in mistaken assumptions about the psychological frailty of people, especially under crisis conditions. I show how these led to a series of policy decisions that limited the containment of virus transmission: the delay in introducing measures at the start of the pandemic; the failure to provide people with support to self-isolate; the lack of community engagement initiatives to increase vaccine roll-out. Finally, I propose that this lack of trust, support and engagement in turn dented the trust that the public had in the Government and in each other — further undermining the pandemic response. I conclude by arguing that a successful response to COVID-19 and to future such events depends upon a fundamental shift in thinking whereby the public are seen as a partner and part of the solution — not the problem — in a crisis.

Introduction

Trust matters. It matters particularly in an emergency, such as the COVID-19 pandemic, where all is unprecedented and uncertain; where we do not fully understand what is going on and how to deal with it; where different sources are telling us different things about what is happening and what to do; where we cannot verify the information given to us by these different sources, we cannot determine what is right and what is wrong from the information alone and therefore all we can go on is our relationship to these different sources. Do we trust what they are telling us or not?

Most of us are not virologists, epidemiologists or modellers. We cannot be expert on how the virus spreads and how to stop it spreading. We cannot independently evaluate how safe and effective vaccines are. We cannot determine whether masks really make a difference. So do we listen to the medical, scientific and Governmental authorities who advise us to take precautions? Or do we heed the sceptics who tell us that there is no real threat and this is nothing but a ruse to control us and remove our freedoms? Trust — and more specifically, who we trust — really does matter.

There is a wealth of evidence that points to the importance of trust. Trust in Government has been shown to lead to a series of COVID outcomes including increasing the perceived fairness of official information about COVID [1], increasing the value of this information [2], lowering infection rates [3] and lowering levels of COVID mortality [4]. However, the most common finding concerns the relationship between trust in Government and increased adherence to COVID regulations and recommendations. This has been shown in countries as diverse as China [5], Ethiopia [6] and France [7].

Bollyky and colleagues [8] take the argument a step further. They argue that, even taking into account other core aspects of a society, such as whether it is democratic or not, high trust in Government plays a major role in determining COVID infection rates. Accordingly, they conclude: "Perhaps this pandemic can be a catalyst for the societal reforms needed to earn and nurture public confidence and social solidarity. COVID-19 has shown that the democracies that can mobilise public trust are best placed to survive and thrive even in the face of great adversity".

This is a powerful rallying cry. And, as the various inquiries and pandemic preparedness committees in different countries work through their agendas, we would do well to remember that the slogan 'Build Back Better' that we heard regularly — at least in the early period of the pandemic — is not just about numbers of hospital beds, provision of personal protective equipment, systems of data surveillance and other aspects of health infrastructure. It must also be about creating more trusting social relations in our society.

But this is a rather broad ambition. The term 'trust' is complex [9] and covers many different types of relationship. Most obviously, we can draw a distinction between the trust people have in each other and the trust which people have in Government. But in this chapter I want to start off on a road more rarely travelled. That is, I shall explore the trust which the Government have in the people. I will focus on the case of the UK and show how a lack of trust on behalf of the British Government, rooted in false assumptions about human psychology, led them to implement (or fail to implement) a series of policy decisions which greatly increased the damage done by COVID. Next, I will examine various ways in which the Government's lack of trust in the public led them to treat people in ways that then led the public to lose trust in the Government and also in each other. I shall conclude by considering what we might learn from these errors and how we can do better in the future.

Distrusting the Public

The Roots of Distrust

I became involved in the UK Government behavioural science advisory group on COVID-19 (SPI-B) through my previous work on public behaviour in emergencies and my participation in a number of official advisory groups addressing this issue. One constant in my experience of these groups was that Governments (of whatever stripe) viewed the public as psychologically flawed, beset by biases and hence unable to deal with complex, uncertain or probabilistic information. It is a conception I have previously described as the 'fragile rationalist' [10].

This conception is exemplified by the Behavioural Insights Team (BIT), more popularly known as the 'Nudge Unit', which was set up in the UK Cabinet Office in 2010 and has had considerable influence in the Government ever since [11]. Their concept of 'nudge', derived from the work of Thaler & Sunstein [12], starts from the premise that people do not know their own minds. Us 'cognitive laggards' (a term used by Mols and colleagues [13] in their extended critique of 'nudge') cannot be reasoned with or persuaded through information. Hence we need to be influenced by altering the choice architecture around us and by making 'desirable' behaviours easier to enact. While certainly there is a considerable role to be played by incentivising beneficial behaviours and discouraging harmful ones, and while it makes eminent sense to make the 'right' thing the easier thing to do, such an approach ignores the importance of the relationship between authorities and the public. Still worse, by treating the public as beyond reason and hence excluding engagement with the public, it runs the danger (as we shall subsequently see) of alienating people from authority.

From the perspective of 'fragile rationalism', cognitive deficiencies are particularly problematic in a crisis. If our ability to think straight is limited at the best of times, put us under pressure and we fall apart. We panic, we lose our rationality entirely and we threaten to turn a crisis into a catastrophe. Hence, in such times (as for instance during a pandemic), the public are very much part of the problem and need to be managed as such. One important aspect of this is the management of information. If you tell people too much about the treats that confront them, they will be all the more likely to panic and run out of control.

These assumptions are sufficiently robust to resist the empirical evidence about behaviour in emergencies. This shows that panic (in the sense of a dysfunctional over-reaction to threat) is extremely rare, that people generally support each other in emergencies (even if they are strangers), and that where disasters do occur it tends to be less a result of psychological dysfunctionality than of environmental factors and failures of management, such as lacking, blocking or even locking exits [14]. Moreover, people are far more likely to die as a result of being given too little information about a threat and how to save themselves from it rather than from too much information [15].

Underpinning the solidarity of people in emergencies is a sense of emergent social identity [16]. That is, the common experience of threat leads people to shift from thinking of themselves in terms of 'I' (personal identity) to 'we' (social identity). Once our sense of self extends to include others, so we begin to be more concerned about them, trust and respect them more, to agree with them more and be influenced by them more, to help and expect to be helped by them more [17]. As we form a psychological group, so we become a more effective co-acting unit with a greater psychological sense of coping and greater practical ability to deal with the challenges we face [18]. Resilience is not something that we do (or do not) have within us as individuals, its limits being brutally exposed in times of crisis. Resilience is something which develops between us in the circumstances of crisis.

These points do not just apply to 'horizontal' relations amongst members of the public. They also apply to 'vertical' relations between public and (Governmental) authorities. To the extent that Government is seen as being of — and acting for — the public, so the public will have greater trust and respect for Government and also will be more likely to accept Government laws, regulations and advice [19].

The implication of this is that the failure of Government to understand the psychology of collectivity and of resilience (and of the relationship between the two) will lead them to underestimate the potential of a unified public as a resource in responding to a crisis. It may also lead them to pursue policies that lose them the support of the public in dealing with the crisis. After all, if you take people for fools and treat them as a problem, you will undermine any notion of common cause they might have had with you and you them [20].

The greater the crisis, the more the dangers of getting the psychology of crisis wrong. And during the COVID-19 pandemic — the greatest crisis of our generation — the limits and the costs of a psychology of distrust were exposed with particular brutality. Let us start by illustrating how such distrust of the public led to tragic policy misjudgements. There are numerous such examples. I only have space to address three of the most egregious.

Behavioural Fatigue

On March 9th, 2020, Italy — with nearly 10,000 COVID-19 cases and almost 500 deaths — announced the introduction of comprehensive quarantine measures ('lockdown'). On that same date, there had only been four deaths in the UK, but cases were rising rapidly and the Government was considering its response. The Chief Medical Officer (CMO) for England, Chris Whitty, said in a live televised briefing: "*Anything we do, we have got to be able to sustain. Once we have started these things we have to continue them through the peak, and there is a risk that, if we go too early, people will understandably get fatigued and it will be difficult to sustain this over time*" (cited in [21]). Three days later, on March 12th, he elaborated this statement, claiming that behavioural science shows what is *"common sense to everybody in this audience"*, namely that *"people start off with the best of intentions, but enthusiasm at a certain point starts to flag"*. In short, individuals lack the ability to stick with tough measures for long so it is best to delay them until they are absolutely necessary.

This notion of 'behavioural fatigue' played a part in delaying the introduction of 'lockdown' measures in the UK until 23rd March, 2020 — possibly by as much as a week [22]. Once lockdown was finally imposed, this 'common sense' notion of behavioural fatigue turned out to be wrong — at least as far as the first wave of the pandemic is concerned. As in previous emergencies, so during COVID-19, people did not panic or fall apart. Levels of adherence to 'lockdown' were extremely high and stayed consistently high over a prolonged period [23] — albeit with a notable exception, which I will consider later. One study showed that less than 10% of people were resisting regulations, even though roughly half of them were suffering considerably (psychologically as well as economically) from doing so [24]. Moreover, when people failed to adhere, it was predominantly due to practical constraints rather than psychologically frailties. Thus Atchison and colleagues [25] showed that vulnerable groups and ethnic minorities were far more likely to break lockdown. Their motivation to stay home was indistinguishable from the more privileged. It was simply that they were unable to both stay home and put food on their family's table.

But it was not just that 'behavioural fatigue' was wrong. It was dangerously and tragically wrong. It has been claimed that delaying lockdown doubled the numbers of infections and deaths in the first wave, costing as many as 30,000 lives [26]. Subsequent modelling [27] suggests that, had lockdown been introduced on the 16th as opposed to the 23rd, cases would have been reduced by as much as 74% and total deaths by 34,000 (and the time spent in full lockdown could have been reduced from 69 to 35 days). Moreover, if the UK had introduced such measures two weeks earlier on the 9th (the day Chris Whitty invoked 'behavioural fatigue'), cases would have been reduced by 93% and deaths by 43,000. In this case, getting the behavioural science wrong was literally a matter of life and death for tens of thousands of people.

So where did the notion of behavioural fatigue come from? Despite the CMO's assertion, it certainly did not come from behavioural scientists themselves. An open letter to the Government on March 16th from 681 behavioural scientists denied that there was an evidence base for 'behavioural fatigue' [28]. The Government's own official behavioural science advisory group, SPI-B, never endorsed the idea and indeed senior participants in the group dismissed it as *"an ill-defined new term that had no basis in behavioural science"* [29]. Some suggest that the notion derived from other sources of behavioural science advice to the Government, notably the BIT (*e.g.,* [30]). However, they themselves subsequently denied that they were the source. The Head of Communications insisted *"absolutely, categorically"* that 'behavioural fatigue' did not come from *"us or anyone at BIT"* [21].

In the end, it is unclear exactly how Chris Whitty arrived at the idea (which was then taken as fact by decision makers). One suggestion is that he derived it from his own experience of people failing to take prescriptions through to completion [22]. However, in the end, it is, perhaps, less important to ask 'who came up with the idea?' than 'why was the idea of behavioural fatigue so quickly embraced and treated as fact by the Prime Minister, the Health Secretary and other key decision makers?'. The answer, I suggest, is that it fits so well with their wider distrust in the psychology of the general public.

Lack of Support

In their 2020 Annual Report, Oxford Languages documented how the COVID-19 pandemic had transformed the English language, introducing a host of new terms, including 'covidiot', defined as 'a person who disobeys guidelines designed to prevent the spread of COVID-19' [31]. The word was in the headlines as early as the first day of the lockdown (before which there were no formal guidelines to disobey), referring to those who left their homes and packed together in country beauty spots and urban parks [32]. The response by many local councils across the UK was either to close parks or else to threaten to do so [33].

The concept of 'covidiots' does more than simply describe the act of disobedience. It explains it through the intellectual and moral failings of the disobedient. They are either too stupid or too selfish to appreciate the consequences of their actions. They deserve condemnation and punishment. Yet the evidence shows that, on both counts, the term is misapplied to most of those to whom it was applied. On the one hand, going out once a day for exercise was allowed within the rules. On the other, of the 20% of people who did break the rules on going out, only 1% or 2% did so 'for fun' and 14–15% did so out of necessity [34]. Moreover, as many pointed out (*e.g.*, [35]), for those living in towns and cities, especially those living in high-rise flats or without gardens, the only places to which they could go out (as allowed) were the parks. And, given the limited number of parks available (and growing more limited due to the privatisation of green spaces in cities like London — see [36]), people could not help but find themselves packed together.

As we argued in a paper from the Scottish Government COVID-19 Advisory Group [37], insofar as the problem of crowding in public arose less from lack of goodwill than lack of space, it is counter-productive to punish people by further restricting the spaces they could use. It would be far more effective to support them by providing more spaces — for instance opening up the facilities that had been privatised, allowing people to use school playing fields or the 48,000 acres of golf courses that exist in London alone.

If the assumption of individual frailty delayed the onset of COVID measures, as soon as measures were implemented, the assumption of frailty contributed to a policy of blame and punishment rather than provision of the support which would enable people to adhere. This approach became more firmly entrenched when the first UK national lockdown was lifted and debate started about local measures in areas of high COVID prevalence, such as Leicester [38].

The Government's advisory group on behaviour, SPI-B, contributed a paper to this debate, which stressed the following points [39]. First, higher levels of prevalence derive from greater exposure to the virus which in turn derives from local living conditions: crowded housing, use of public transport, poor health and safety at work and public-facing jobs. Hence, prevalence is more a function of deprivation than of (mis)behaviour. Second, any measures that are introduced must therefore be accompanied by wide-ranging packages of support, because "*without targeted support, pre-existing inequalities may make adherence impossible*". Third, it is important more generally to frame interventions as supportive, as designed "***with and for***" the local community (emphasis in the original) rather than "*something that is done **to** people*" (ditto). This extends to the very language with which interventions are described. More specifically, there is a need for "*curtailing the use of the punitive and stigmatising term 'lockdown'*" and instead using terms that "*emphasise care, concern and support for the affected communities*".

This advice was largely ignored. The language of lockdown became almost universally employed to describe COVID measures and, more seriously, measures were not accompanied by the support necessary for people — especially members of deprived groups — to abide by them. This was true both in terms of support for local Government — leading to their opposition to the introduction of measures [40] — and also in terms of support for individuals.

Probably the most egregious failure to support individuals relates to the requirement for those who are infected with COVID-19 to self-isolate. This is far more onerous than other measures — such as wearing masks or keeping one's distance from others. For many it involves an unsustainable loss of income, for many more (especially those living in crowded multi-generation households) it raises insoluble practical problems. As noted [41], without support — especially financial support — self-isolation is all but impossible. Despite this, the Government limited provision to a maximum £500 payment for which only one in eight workers were even eligible to apply, and of those who did apply, seven in ten were rejected [42]. They did not even consider broader 'wrap around' packages of support (providing everything from hotel accommodation to dog walking) as introduced in many other places from Kerala to New York [43].

The consequence was that self-isolation was the one exception (alluded to above) to generally high levels of adherence to COVID measures. While different studies produce somewhat different figures, roughly half or less of the population fully isolated themselves as required [43]. What is more, there is evidence that the financial and practical burdens problems of self-isolation did not only affect what people did once infected but also discouraged them from even getting tested. They simply could not afford to find out that they were unwell [44].

So why were the Government so resolute in refusing to provide support for self-isolation? On 10th June 2021 the then Health Secretary, Matt Hancock, was asked precisely that question when appearing before the joint Science & Technology and Health & Social Care Committees of the House of Commons. He replied: "*The challenge that we had with that proposal is the extent to which it might be gamed*" [45]. In other words, and from the horse's mouth, the Government failed to give people the support they needed to adhere to COVID measures because they did not trust them to act responsibly.

Vaccine Hesitancy

The development of COVID vaccines and their introduction in December 2020 was clearly a game changer in the history of the pandemic. However, it did not render behavioural issues irrelevant. Rather it put a set of new behavioural issues on the agenda — most obviously how to get people to get vaccinated. While, at a general population level, vaccine hesitancy was low, it was much higher in specific communities. Thus, for instance, data collected in the UK at the time the roll-out began found an overall hesitancy figure of 18%. But it was 21% in women, 27% in 16–24 year olds, and as high as 72% amongst Black British respondents [46].

When it comes to explaining hesitancy, there is, as Vanderslott and colleagues document, a longstanding tradition in many countries of attributing it to public ignorance — a stance, they argue, which conveniently serves to blame the people rather than the Government for low vaccine uptake [47]. There is equally a long history in the UK of blaming the public for the failure of vaccination programs [48], and this was equally apparent during the COVID pandemic. The Cabinet Office Minister, Michael Gove, described those who refused the vaccine as 'selfish' [49], while another minister branded them as 'idiots' [50]. Correspondingly, the debate over how to increase vaccination rates centred on whether to restrict the unvaccinated by making 'vaccine passports' a condition of entry to pubs, clubs and other public facilities [51].

Riley-Smith and Donnelly [50] record that others in the Government (such as the then Business Secretary, Kwasi Kwarteng) challenged such explanations and warned against 'stigmatising' those who did not get vaccinated. After initially announcing plans, the UK Government eventually ditched the introduction of vaccine passports [52]. Nonetheless, once again a debate centred on individual deficits — whatever its outcome — served to distract from a consideration of group processes and of relationships between groups. Indeed, the most obvious problem with describing the unvaccinated as stupid or selfish is that it cannot account for the very stark group differences in take-up (unless one wants to go down the very dangerous path of claiming that certain groups are lacking in intellect or morality).

These groups are predominantly ones with a troubled history of relationships to, and trust in, authority. This includes medical authorities. Black Britons in particular can point to a number of historical examples of medical abuse

[53], and a recent report from a joint committee of the House of Commons and the House of Lords shows that 60% of black Britons (roughly the same proportion shown to be vaccine hesitant) believe that the National Health Service does not protect their health to the same degree as white people [54].

What is more, amongst both individuals and populations who are suspicious of the vaccine, the introduction of vaccine passports — especially for everyday activities — is seen as an act of coercion, further eroding their relationship with those advocating vaccination, and decreasing vaccination intentions [55]. In other words, vaccine passports run the danger of alienating the very people who need to be won over.

But again, the real importance of the vaccine passport debate lay in how it stole attention from what we should have been debating — namely how to develop a community engagement strategy as a means of improving vaccine uptake, especially amongst marginalised communities [53]. Such a strategy should, according to the WHO [56], be 'at the centre' of vaccine introduction programs, and has proved highly effective across a range of contexts [57], including the current pandemic in the UK [58]. Its purpose is precisely to work with, rather than impose on, communities. It is rooted in partnership: going to people rather than waiting for them to come to you; communicating through community leaders, listening to and respecting people's concerns rather than treating them as irrational. It is fundamentally about creating an ingroup relationship — the psychological underpinning of trust — with historically marginalised groups.

While there are many excellent local examples of community engagement being used to improve vaccination take-up amongst Black and other marginalised groups in the UK (*e.g.*, [59]), there was no concerted national approach. Here again, a proven strategy rooted in partnership was marginalised due to ingrained assumptions about the psychological frailty of the public.

Sewing Division

Thus far, I have concentrated on the way in which the Government's lack of trust in the public led to a series of policy decisions which undermined the UK response to COVID-19. However, in passing (and notably with regard to vaccination), we have also seen how Government lack of trust had a more indirect (but still important) impact on the COVID response by impacting on public trust and thereby on the behaviour of the public. This can be divided into two distinct processes: the impact of Government actions on what I have previously termed vertical relations (the trust the public have in Government) and the impact on horizontal relations (the trust the public have in each other).

I shall (briefly) deal with each of these in turn.

Vertical Trust

The issue of trust in Government during the pandemic has been dominated by the question of the Government breaking its own rules — starting with Dominic Cummings (the Prime Minister's advisor) travelling to Durham and Barnard Castle. Certainly this was associated with a sharp decline in trust in the UK Government, in contrast to trust in other UK administrations [60]. However, it is instructive to consider why. As Jonathon Rentoul wrote when stories of Downing Street parties began to break: "The most damaging perception of the government throughout the pandemic is that it passed laws that it didn't abide by itself". Or, in more colloquial terms, the Government's actions replaced the initial view that 'we're all in it together' with a shared perception that there was 'one rule for us, another for them' [61].

As I have already pointed out, as the sense of shared identity gives way to a division into ingroup and outgroup, so we become alienated from authority and more resistant to its messages and demands. Certainly, applying different rules to different people is a powerful way of dividing those people into separate groups, but it is far from the only way. The literature on 'procedural justice' shows that the way authorities treat people — whether they listen to us, take account of us, respect us — has a powerful impact on whether we view these authorities as 'us' or 'them' [62].

From this perspective, one could not do worse than to start by positioning the public as a problem and hence as an 'other' which Government needs to manage. All that flows from such a positioning — lack of dialogue and listening, pathologising language, blame for rising infection levels — then contributes to alienating the public from authority. But the problems are perhaps best encapsulated in the use of punishments for those breaking COVID regulations. Both the SPI-B [63] and the SPI-B Policing & Security Sub-Group [64] produced papers which warned against the use of fines and other sanctions for those in breach. They pointed to the lack of evidence for the effectiveness of such sanctions. They challenged the underlying assumption that people who break the rules do so out of lack of motivation to adhere and highlighted the evidence that the key issue is lack of resources. They stressed that penalising those who cannot help breaking the rules is likely to increase tension with the enforcing authorities and undermine their legitimacy. They stressed that the dangers are particularly stark in marginal and deprived communities where resource issues are more acute. The Policing & Security Sub-Group was particularly blunt in warning that "in localities in which relations between communities are already poor, this may also prove combustible" [64]. At worst, then, the lack of trust which the Government has in the public will not just undermine any trust that the public has in the Government. It may lead to open conflict [65].

Horizontal Trust

When Government focus on individual violations of COVID rules, and when they place blame on individuals for those violations, they do not just undermine our relationship with themselves. They also undermine our relationships with each other. For, while we may consider such blame to be inaccurate and unfair when it applies to ourselves, we are more likely to accept it when applied to others. After all, while we can always observe ourselves, by and large we cannot observe directly what the rest of the population are doing. As a consequence, our estimates are greatly influenced by what we are told by politicians as filtered through and amplified by the media — and the media are more likely to lead on stories of raves, parties and other violations than the mundane reality of people staying in, sitting on the sofa and watching TV.

Such an 'availability effect' [66] leads people to the belief that, while they are adhering themselves, others are not. It explains the striking finding that, in 2020, 92% of people evaluated their own adherence as higher than average, and only 2% thought it lower [67]. It also has a series of toxic consequences.

First, if we are led to believe that the norm in our communities is one of non-adherence, then we are less likely to adhere ourselves [68]– either because we see little point in doing so or because we are less sure it is the right thing to do. But even if we ourselves believe in doing something (such as following

COVID regulations), we are less likely to do it if we see others as opposed to it [69].

Second, if people are led to believe that the COVID threat is driven by major violations of the rules — such as large raves and house parties which received so much attention from both Government and media [70] — they are liable to discount the relevance of their own, more minor, violations. So, for instance, in the week when the BBC website carried the headline 'COVID in Scotland: Police break up hundreds of parties every week', figures from Police Scotland recorded that only 12 out of their 279 COVID-related callouts were for gatherings involving 15 or more people. The great majority of violations involved people having one or two more people around than the six then permissible [71]. What is more, senior commanders told me that, when their officers knocked on the door of these households, they were generally met with bemusement if not hostility. People told them that they should be out stopping raves rather than harassing ordinary people who were doing nothing wrong!

Third, if we are led to believe that neighbours are violating rules and are thereby putting us at greater risk of infection, we are likely to begin to view them with suspicion — all the more so when the police and the Government set up hotlines encouraging people to report on others who were breaking regulations or else fraudulently claiming COVID benefits [72]. In a context where adherence and non-adherence were being moralised (the former being 'good people' and the latter 'bad people' who break the rules out of selfishness or stupidity), it is likely to exacerbate neighbourhood tensions [73] and contribute to rising levels of anger and confrontation amongst the public [74].

While this is toxic enough in itself, it becomes considerably more dangerous if the moral categories of adherence and non-adherence are mapped onto existing lines of social division, especially those of ethnicity and 'race'. Thus, if the higher rates of infection, hospitalisation and death amongst ethnic minorities [75] are blamed on the members of those minorities themselves — and still worse, if those minorities are then blamed for the pandemic amongst majority group members, then the conditions are created for intergroup hatred [76].

While the pandemic did lead to increases in hate crimes, especially against people of Chinese origin (Chelsea & Hansen, in press), it has not led to the level of ethnic violence seen historically in pandemics such as the persecution of Jews during the Black Death [77], which reached its height in incidents such as the massacre of some 2,000 people in Strasbourg on St Valentine's Day,

1349 [78]. However, it is important not to be complacent. If COVID were to become a disease embedded in marginalised communities due to deprivation and alienation, and if it had the potential to flare up in the wider society, then these toxic histories have every chance of repeating themselves.

Conclusion

Throughout this chapter, I have argued for the importance of trust as part of a successful societal response to the pandemic, for the importance of shared identity (a sense of community) to the creation of trust (and of trust to the creation of shared identity) and therefore, for the need to understand the collective psychology of community building. If you get that right, and are able to bring authorities and communities together, then the public can become a partner in responding to the pandemic. They will help the authorities and each other in surmounting even the most challenging times. They will be your most valuable resource.

Sadly, however, I have had to develop that story in the breach, by recounting how the UK Government failed to understand the importance of trust and, through its distrust of the public, made disastrous policy choices, lost the trust of the public and eroded the trust of the public in each other. Seeing the public as a problem not only stopped them becoming a resource but actually turned them into a problem.

There are three general lessons to be taken from this.

The first is that we need to be sanguine about the psychology of groups, neither treating it as all bad nor as all good. Much depends upon the way we draw boundaries. When groups are inclusive and everybody is viewed as part of 'us', then the sense of shared identity can give rise to trust, solidarity and resilience. However, when the psychology of 'us' gives way to that of 'us' and 'them' — and where, moreover, those who are not of 'us' are seen as a problem for 'us' — then the sense of threatened identity can give rise to mistrust, suspicion and fragmentation. Like dynamite, groups are powerful. But whether they are powerful for construction or destruction depends on understanding their potential and treating them with considerable care.

The second lesson, which flows from this, is that behavioural science is every bit as powerful as medical science in dealing with a pandemic. But power is a mixed blessing, because it comes with accountability. Getting the psychology right (or wrong) is no longer an academic exercise. It becomes, quite literally, a matter of life and death. As we have seen, in getting the psychology wrong, the Government cost us an awful lot of lives.

Third — and to conclude as I began — let us recall how, early on in the pandemic, there was a lot of talk of using the insights we gained from COVID to 'build back better'. An essential part of that is to appreciate the importance of trust and community and to gain a better understanding of their psychology so as better to build them (or, at a minimum, so as not to destroy them). We must not make the same mistakes next time round.

References

[1] Han, Q, Zheng, B, Cristea, M, Agostini, M, Bélanger, JJ, Gützkow, B, Krienenkamp, J, PsyCorona Team & Leander, P (2021). Trust in government regarding COVID-19 and its associations with preventive health behaviour and prosocial behaviour during the pandemic: a cross-sectional and longitudinal study. *Psychological Medicine*, **51**, 1–11.

[2] Fridman, I, Lucas, N, Henke, D, & Zigler, CK (2020). Association between public knowledge about COVID-19, trust in information sources, and adherence to social distancing: cross-sectional survey. *JMIR Public Health and Surveillance*, **6**(3), e22060.

[3] Ye, M & Lyu, Z (2020). Trust, risk perception, and COVID-19 infections: Evidence from multilevel analyses of combined original dataset in China. *Social Science and Medicine*, **265**, 113517.

[4] Farzanegan, MR & Hofmann, HP (2022). A matter of trust? Political trust and the COVID-19 pandemic. *International Journal of Sociology*, **52**(6), 476–499.

[5] Min, C, Shen, F, Yu, W & Chu, Y (2020). The relationship between government trust and preventive behaviors during the COVID-19 pandemic in China: exploring the roles of knowledge and negative emotion. *Preventive Medicine*, **141**, 106288.

[6] Shanka, MS & Menebo, MM (2022). When and how trust in Government leads to compliance with Covid-19 precautionary measures. *Journal of Business Research*, **139**, 1275–1283.

[7] Raude, J, Lecrique, JM, Lasbeur, L, Leon, C, Guignard, R, Du Roscoät, E & Arwidson, P (2020). Determinants of preventive behaviors in response to the COVID-19 pandemic in France: Comparing the sociocultural, psychosocial, and social cognitive explanations. *Frontiers in Psychology*, **11**, 584500.

[8] Bollyky, TJ, Angelino, O, Wigley, S & Dieleman, JL (2022). Trust made the difference for democracies in COVID-19. *The Lancet*, **400**(10353), 657.

[9] Simpson, JA (2007). Psychological foundations of trust. *Current Directions in Psychological Science*, **16**(5), 264–268.

[10] Reicher, SD & Bauld, L (2021). From the 'fragile rationalist' to 'collective resilience': what human psychology has taught us about the Covid-19 pandemic and what the

Covid-19 pandemic has taught us about human psychology. *Journal of the Royal College of Physicians of Edinburgh*, **51**(1_suppl), 12–19.

[11] James, S (2015). The contribution of the UK's behavioural insights team. *International Journal of Applied Behavioral Economics*, **4**(2), 53–70.

[12] Thaler, RH & Sunstein, CR (2009). *Nudge: Improving Decisions about Health, Wealth, and Happiness*. Penguin.

[13] Mols, F, Haslam, SA, Jetten, J & Steffens, NK (2015). Why a nudge is not enough: A social identity critique of governance by stealth. *European Journal of Political Research*, **54**(1), 81–98.

[14] Drury, J (2018). The role of social identity processes in mass emergency behaviour: An integrative review. *European Review of Social Psychology*, **29**(1), 38–81.

[15] Drury, J, Reicher, SD & Stott, C (2020). COVID-19 in context: Why do people die in emergencies? It's probably not because of collective psychology. *British Journal of Social Psychology*, **59**(3), 686–693.

[16] Drury, J (2012). Collective Resilience in Mass Emergencies and Disasters: A Social Identity Model. In Jetten, J, Haslam, C & Haslam, SA (Eds.), *The Social Cure*, pp. 195–215. Psychology Press.

[17] Reicher, SD & Haslam, SA (2009). Beyond Help. In Sturmer, S & Snyder, M (Eds.), *The Psychology of Prosocial Behavior: Group Processes, Intergroup Relations, and Helping*, pp. 289–309. Blackwell.

[18] Drury, J & Reicher, SD (2020). Crowds and Collective Behaviour. In Hogg, M (Ed.), *Oxford Research Encyclopedia of Psychology*. Oxford University Press.

[19] Tyler, TR (2006). *Why People Obey the Law*. Princeton University Press.

[20] Turner, JC (1991). *Social Influence*. Open University Press.

[21] Mahase, E (2020). Covid-19: Was the decision to delay the UK's lockdown over fears of "behavioural fatigue" based on evidence?. *BMJ*, **370**, m3166.

[22] Conn, D, Lawrence, F, Lewis, P, Carrell, S, Pegg, D, Davies, H & Evens, R (2020, April 29). Revealed: the inside story of the UK's Covid-19 crisis. *The Guardian*. www.theguardian.com/world/2020/apr/29/revealed-the-inside-story-of-uk-covid-19-coronavirus-crisis.

[23] Reicher, SD & Drury, J (2021). Pandemic fatigue? How adherence to covid-19 regulations has been misrepresented and why it matters. *BMJ*, **372**, n137.

[24] Duffy, B & Allington, D (2020). The accepting, the suffering, and the resisting: the different reactions to life under lockdown. *Policy Institute, King's College London*. www.kcl.ac.uk/policy-institute/assets/Coronavirus-in-the-UK-cluster-analysis.pdf.

[25] Atchison, C, Bowman, LR, Vrinten, C, Redd, R, Pristerà, P, Eaton, J & Ward, H (2021). Early perceptions and behavioural responses during the COVID-19 pandemic: a cross-sectional survey of UK adults. *BMJ Open*, **11**(1), e043577.

[26] Buchan, L (2020, June 10). Lockdown one week earlier could have halved UK's death toll, says ex-government scientist. *The Independent*. https://www.independent.co.uk/news/uk/politics/uk-lockdown-coronavirus-death-toll-neil-ferguson-a9559051.html.

[27] Arnold, KF, Gilthorpe, MS, Alwan, NA, Heppenstall, AJ, Tomova, GD, McKee, M & Tennant, PW (2022). Estimating the effects of lockdown timing on COVID-19 cases and deaths in England: A counterfactual modelling study. *Plos One*, **17**(4), e0263432.

[28] Hahn, U, *et al.* (2020, March 16). Open letter to the UK Government regarding COVID-19. https://sites.google.com/view/covidopenletter/home.

[29] Michie, S & West, R (2020). Behavioural, environmental, social, and systems interventions against Covid-19. *BMJ*, **370**, m2982.

[30] Hutton, R (2020, March 10). Keep calm and wash your hands. Britain's strategy to beat Virus. *Bloomberg UK*. https://www.bloomberg.com/news/articles/2020-03-11/keep-calm-and-wash-your-hands-britain-s-strategy-to-beat-virus?leadSource=uverify%20wall.

[31] Oxford Languages (2020). 2020: Words of an unprecedented year. *Oxford University Press*. https://v.fastcdn.co/u/2014a5b7/54382502-0-Words-of-an-Unpreced.pdf.

[32] Dixon, H (2020, March 23). Rural residents tell visitors to go home, with parks and beauty spots packed. *The Telegraph*. https://www.telegraph.co.uk/news/2020/03/22/rural-residents-tell-visitors-go-home-parks-beauty-spots-packed/.

[33] De Castella, T (2020, March 23). Ministers leave it to Councils to decide on park closures. *Local Government Chronicle*. https://www.lgcplus.com/politics/coronavirus/parks-closed-across-country-in-bid-to-enforce-social-distancing-23-03-2020/.

[34] Coronavirus daily tracker: 23rd March — 2nd April 2020 (2020). *YouGov*. https://docs.cdn.yougov.com/412s271exg/YouGov%20-%20Daily%20coronavirus%20tracker%2023%20Mar%20-%205%20Apr.pdf.

[35] Fairs, M (2020, April 6). Architects lead backlash over park closures and "heavy handed" policing in London's open spaces. *DeZeen*. https://www.dezeen.com/2020/04/06/backlash-park-closure-london-brockwell-park/.

[36] Shenker, J (2017, July 24). Revealed: the insidious creep of pseudo-public space in London. *The Guardian*. https://www.theguardian.com/cities/2017/jul/24/revealed-pseudo-public-space-pops-london-investigation-map.

[37] Reicher, SD, Stott, C, Drury, J, Amlot, R, Bear, L, Bennell, C, *et al.* (2020). Facilitating adherence to social distancing measures during the Covid-19 pandemic. *Scottish Government Covid-19 Advisory Group*. https://www.gov.scot/binaries/content/documents/govscot/publications/research-and-analysis/2020/06/covid-19-advisory-group-evidence-papers-april-2020/documents/facilitating-adherence-to-social-distancing-measures-during-the-covid-19-pandemic-15-april-2020/facilitating-adherence-to-social-distancing-measures-during-the-covid-19-pandemic-15-april-2020/govscot%3Adocument/Facilitating%2Badherence%2Bto%2Bsocial%2Bdistancing%2Bmeasures%2Bduring%2Bthe%2BCOVID%2B19%2Bpandemic%2B%2528 15%2BApril%2B2020%2529.pdf.

[38] Hancock, M (2020, June 29). Plans for managing the coronavirus (COVID-19) outbreak in Leicester. *GOV.UK*. https://www.gov.uk/government/speeches/local-action-to-tackle-coronavirus.

[39] SPI-B (2020, July 29). Consensus statement on local interventions. *GOV.UK*. https://www.gov.uk/government/publications/spi-b-consensus-statement-on-local-interventions-29-july-2020/spi-b-consensus-statement-on-local-interventions-29-july-2020.

[40] Blackall, M (2020, October 10). North of England mayors reject support plans for local Covid lockdowns. *The Guardian*. https://www.theguardian.com/world/2020/oct/10/north-of-england-mayors-reject-support-package-for-local-covid-lockdowns.

[41] SPI-B (2020, September 16). The impact of financial and other targeted support on rates of self-isolation or quarantine. *GOV.UK*. https://assets.publishing.service.gov.uk/government/uploads/system/uploads/attachment_data/file/925133/S0759_SPI-B__The_impact_of_financial_and_other_targeted_support_on_rates_of_self-isolation_or_quarantine_.pdf.

[42] Collinson, A (2021, February 15). High rejection rates show the self-isolation payment scheme isn't fit for purpose. *TUC*. https://www.tuc.org.uk/blogs/high-rejection-rates-show-self-isolation-payment-scheme-isnt-fit-purpose.

[43] Reicher, SD, Drury, J & Michie, S (2021, April 5). Contrasting figures on adherence to self-isolation show that support is even more important than ever. *British Medical Journal*. https://blogs.bmj.com/bmj/2021/04/05/why-contrasting-figures-on-adherence-to-self-isolation-show-that-support-to-self-isolate-is-even-more-important-than-we-previously-realised/.

[44] Liverpool Covid-SMART community testing pilot: evaluation report (2021, June 17). *University of Liverpool*. https://www.liverpool.ac.uk/media/livacuk/research/Mass,testing,evaluation.pdf.

[45] Science and Technology Committee, Health and Social Care Committee. Oral evidence: coronavirus: lessons learnt, HC 95 (2021, June 10). *UK Parliament*. https://committees.parliament.uk/oralevidence/2318/pdf/.

[46] Robertson, E, *et al.* (2021). Predictors of COVID-19 vaccine hesitancy in the UK household longitudinal study. *Brain, Behavior, and Immunity*, **94**, 41–50.

[47] Vanderslott, S, Enria, L, Bowmer, A, Kamara, A & Lees, S (2022). Attributing public ignorance in vaccination narratives. *Social Science & Medicine*, **307**, 115152.

[48] Millward, G (2019). *Vaccinating Britain: Mass Vaccination and the Public since the Second World War*. Manchester University Press.

[49] Covid: Turning down Covid vaccine is selfish, says Michael Gove (2021, July 27). *BBC News*. https://www.bbc.co.uk/news/uk-politics-57987016.

[50] Riley-Smith, B & Donnelly, L (2021, May 17). People who refuse Covid vaccine are selfish says Lord Lloyd Webber. *The Telegraph*. https://www.telegraph.co.uk/politics/2021/05/17/people-refuse-covid-vaccine-selfish-says-andrew-lloyd-webber/.

[51] Vaughan, A (2021). UK vaccine passport row. *New Scientist*, **250**(3329), 7.

[52] Jackson, M (2021, September 12). England vaccine passport plans ditched, Sajid Javid says. *BBC News*. https://www.bbc.co.uk/news/uk-58535258.

[53] Burgess, RA, *et al.* (2021). The COVID-19 vaccines rush: participatory community engagement matters more than ever. *The Lancet*, **397**(10268), 8–10.

[54] Joint Committee on Human Rights (2020). Black people, racism and human rights. Eleventh report of session 2019–21. *UK Parliament.* https://committees.parliament.uk/publications/3376/documents/32359/default/.

[55] de Figueiredo, A, Larson, HJ & Reicher, SD (2021). The potential impact of vaccine passports on inclination to accept COVID-19 vaccinations in the United Kingdom: Evidence from a large cross-sectional survey and modeling study. *eClinicalMedicine*, **40**, 101109.

[56] Conducting community engagement for COVID-19 vaccines: Interim Guidance (2021). *WHO.* https://apps.who.int/iris/handle/10665/339451.

[57] Nutbeam, D (2021), The vital role of meaningful community engagement in responding to the COVID-19 pandemic. *Public Health Research and Practice*, **31**(1), e3112101.

[58] Hussain, B, Latif, A, Timmons, S, Nkhoma, K & Nellums, LB (2022). Overcoming COVID-19 vaccine hesitancy among ethnic minorities: A systematic review of UK studies. *Vaccine*, **40**(25), 3413–3432.

[59] COVID-19 vaccine hesitancy — debunking the myths using a community engagement approach underpinned by NICE Guidance (2021). *National Institute for Health and Care Excellence.* https://www.nice.org.uk/sharedlearning/covid-19-vaccine-hesitancy-debunking-the-myths-using-a-community-engagement-approach-underpinned-by-nice-guidance.

[60] Fancourt, D, Steptoe, A & Wright, L (2020). The Cummings effect: politics, trust, and behaviours during the COVID-19 pandemic. *The Lancet*, **396**(10249), 464–465.

[61] Rentoul, J (2021, December 16). Once again, it's one rule for us and another rule for them. *The Independent.* https://www.independent.co.uk/voices/boris-johnson-lockdown-party-downing-street-b1977490.html.

[62] Tyler, TR & Blader, SL (2003). The group engagement model: Procedural justice, social identity, and cooperative behavior. *Personality and Social Psychology Review*, **7**(4), 349–361.

[63] SPI-B (2020, April 1). Easing restrictions on activity and social distancing. *GOV.UK.* https://assets.publishing.service.gov.uk/government/uploads/system/uploads/attachment_data/file/884013/28-easing-restrictions-on-activity-and-social-distancing-comments-suggestions-spi-b-01042020.pdf.

[64] SPI-B Security & Policing Sub-Group (2020, September 21). COVID-19 security and policing challenges. *GOV.UK.* https://assets.publishing.service.gov.uk/government/uploads/system/uploads/attachment_data/file/1012400/S0781_SPI-B_PS_Security_and_Policing_Challenges_-_Horizon_Scanning.pdf.

[65] Reicher, S & Stott, C (2020). On order and disorder during the COVID-19 pandemic. *British Journal of Social Psychology*, **59**(3), 694–702.

[66] Tversky, A & Kahneman, D (1973). Availability: A heuristic for judging frequency and probability. *Cognitive Psychology*, **5**, 207–232.

[67] Majority feel they comply with Covid-19 rules better than others (2020, December 4). *UCL News.* https://www.ucl.ac.uk/news/2020/dec/majority-feel-they-comply-covid-19-rules-better-others.

[68] Bonell, C, Michie, S, Reicher, S, West, R, Bear, L, Yardley, L, *et al.* (2020). Harnessing behavioural science in public health campaigns to maintain 'social distancing' in response to the COVID-19 pandemic: key principles. *Journal of Epidemiology and Community Health*, **74**(8), 617–619.

[69] Bonell, C, Michie, S, Reicher, S, West, R, Bear, L, Yardley, L, *et al.* (2020). Harnessing behavioural science in public health campaigns to maintain 'social distancing' in response to the COVID-19 pandemic: key principles. *Journal of Epidemiology and Community Health*, **74**(8), 617–619.

[70] PA Media (2020, August 22). Illegal rave organisers in England face fines of up to £10,000. *The Guardian.* https://www.theguardian.com/world/2020/aug/22/illegal-rave-organisers-in-england-face-fines-of-up-to-10000.

[71] Reicher, SD (2020, November 4). Blaming Covid 'rule-breakers' is a distraction: support is needed, not fines. *The Guardian.* https://www.theguardian.com/commentisfree/2020/nov/04/blaming-covid-rule-breakers-support-fines-lockdown.

[72] New hotline launched to report COVID fraudsters (2020, October 13). *GOV.UK.* https://www.gov.uk/government/news/new-hotline-launched-to-report-covid-fraudsters.

[73] Prosser, AM, Judge, M, Bolderdijk, JW, Blackwood, L & Kurz, T (2020). 'Distancers' and 'non-distancers'? The potential social psychological impact of moralizing COVID-19 mitigating practices on sustained behaviour change. *British Journal of Social Psychology*, **59**(3), 653–662.

[74] Duffy, B (2020). Coronavirus conflict: how the pandemic has fuelled anger and confrontation. *Health Protection Research Unit in Emergency Preparedness and Response, Kings College London.* https://www.kcl.ac.uk/policy-institute/assets/coronavirus-conflict.pdf.

[75] Raleigh, VS (2022). Ethnic differences in Covid-19 death rates. *BMJ*, **376**, o427.

[76] Reicher, S, Haslam, SA & Rath, R (2008). Making a virtue of evil: A five-step social identity model of the development of collective hate. *Social and Personality Psychology Compass*, **2**(3), 1313–1344.

[77] Cohn Jr, SK (2007). The Black Death and the burning of Jews. *Past and Present*, **196**(1), 3–36.

[78] Landau, L (n.d.). La massacre de la Saint-Valentin. *Le judaïsme d'Alsace et de Lorraine — ASIJA.* http://judaisme.sdv.fr/histoire/antisem/peste/stval.htm.

Chapter

8

Navigating the Waves of Change: Emotional Agility as the Compass for Internal Auditors

By Ana Martins and Narishaa Shah

Summary

The coronavirus (COVID-19) pandemic altered many workforce environments, driving almost a forceful directive for employees to work from home. Such a shift in workforce dynamics had many ripple effects on private and public sector businesses and employees. The Internal Audit Unit, that provides internal audit assurance and consulting activities on risk, control and governance processes, at the eThekwini Municipality in Durban, KwaZulu-Natal, South Africa, had compelled its leadership to start looking differently at how internal audit operates and conducts work as a professional unit within the municipality. Having to work under such conditions affected many aspects within the work environment; hence the department had seen the need to assess its working environment, allowing staff to work remotely to ensure it maintained its effectiveness and productivity whilst keeping its employees safe during the various lockdown levels declared by the president of South Africa. This chapter sets out a study of how internal auditors in the South African context have had to harness their emotional agility in order to embrace working remotely as a consequence of COVID-19. The factors considered in this chapter can be used as a benchmark for other internal audit entities to consider in their employee management and remote working strategy. Although the current pandemic of COVID-19 through the various lockdown levels have been restricting workers to come to their offices, the long-term sustainability of internal auditors in bringing innovation and creative solutions to its clients is essential and by evaluating their main resource (employees), based on continuous engagements, commitment levels from employees, and the development of skills, it will better equip the unit on areas for improvement.

Introduction

The COVID-19 global pandemic, acknowledged by the WHO in February 2020, placed all businesses, both private and public, under innumerable challenges. The focus for most organisations is based on their ability to move forward with agility and resilience. Organisational leaders are thinking very long and hard about the turnaround recovery strategies and change in business operations to ensure continued organisational existence and to address unprecedented fiscal setbacks. New opportunities are being sought to better position organisations in delivering effectively and efficiently and to leverage out of redundancy or, worse, becoming obsolete. The pandemic has put a new spotlight on the public sector as citizens and the private sectors turn to governments for guidance, assistance, and information. The eThekwini Municipality, along with all its umbrella of disciplines and units which include the Internal Audit Unit (IAU), is no different. This has left the City Manager, Deputy City Managers, and unit heads with the responsibility of deciding how this transformation will take place and the implications it may have.

The IAU at the eThekwini Municipality had, since the first lockdown announcement in March 2020, seen the need to assess its working environment and has taken steps to allow staff to work remotely to ensure it maintains its effectiveness and productivity whilst keeping its employees safe during the various lockdown levels declared by the president. This crisis had forced the IAU leadership to start looking differently at the way in which it operates and conducts work as a professional unit within the municipality. The pandemic had served as a catalyst in presenting the unit with the opportunity to really assess its processes and start implementing changes to transform the way in which it works, allowing audit teams more flexibility and yet still meeting the requirements of the Institute of Internal Auditing Standards.

The pandemic created the necessity to work from home and resulted in the IAU making the necessary changes to equip employees to ensure continuation of productivity. The changing working environment led to challenges but also presented it with immense opportunities to modernise and embrace current best-in-the-world work environments. This chapter provides insight towards understanding how IAU management perceives the value derived from remote working employees through three main constructs of emotional agility that affect productivity, namely, employee engagement, commitment, and development.

The "new norm", where individuals are required to keep their distance and wear masks continuously since the start of the pandemic, has catapulted the IAU to work remotely and still retain the provision of its services to its client, namely, the eThekwini Municipality. Whilst success has been met on key deliverables, pertinent factors such as employee engagements, commitment levels, and development of the professionals within the unit, it was also important for these to be closely monitored and assessed. Organisational leaders cannot assume that the culture that exists in a traditional office workspace can automatically work in a virtual working environment [1].

It is imperative that the IAU makes informed decisions on the employee's well-being through understanding the implications of employee engagements, commitment, and development during remote working. Lack of this understanding could result in them making inadequate and uninformed decisions that may hinder employee progress, resulting in lost opportunities of human capital investment nurturing the long-term sustainability of employee growth and development in the internal audit profession where human capital is seen as the primary functioning source of a successful IAU. One of the objectives of this work was to evaluate how the factors of emotional agility such as employee engagement, commitment, and development affect the IAU's productivity during remote working. Internal audit by its profession is expected to guide its client base on the remote working factors to consider and set an example on how to start the first step in shifting to a more versatile, agile environment. The unit's investments in its resources are its main source of service provision. Therefore, a study was conducted to assist the IAU to promote emotional agility such as employee communication, commitment, and development during remote working so that internal audit adds value to the eThekwini Municipality in its ability to become more agile, navigating the wave of change. It is expected to offer an informed view on how the leadership of the IAU of the eThekwini Municipality can consider remote working as a new working norm, setting it up to become a more versatile and agile environment for not just the current lockdown circumstances but as the long-term sustainable working solution in the future.

A Review of the Literature

Extant literature is reviewed in this section to provide the framework for the chapter.

Emotional Agility as a Compass

Emotional agility can be described as one's ability to deal with his/her emotions and thoughts that will either change or retain behaviours so that one can live in ways that align to one's goals, values and intentions [2, 3]. The term has not been used widely but is essential to understand as it plays a significant role in one's life for successful survival, especially during volatile and stressful times [3].

Agile employees means that employees are willing to adapt to their environments and make it a success. In order to have sustainable economic growth and a productive employment base, employers need to understand their employee's emotional agility on the human capital elements of communication (social), development (intellectual), and commitment (emotional and spiritual). Whilst many emotions and thoughts can be explored on an employee's behaviour in the workplace, the study included in this chapter focuses on three specific constructs that influence emotional agility of internal auditors during remote working, which are communication, commitment and development. The aim of this study was to garner a deeper understanding of employee emotions and thoughts through these human capital elements to see if such a goal can still be achieved during remote working by internal auditors.

Remote Working and Communication in Internal Auditing

Due to non-visibility in the workplace of employees, there is an increase on employee cynicism and mistrust [4]. The demands placed on employees are greater and hence they have taken on longer hours of work and more responsibility [4]. Individuals are becoming more frustrated and dissatisfied with work, but the "connection" of an individual with organisational outcomes is necessary during these conditions of remote working [4]. The text concludes that Employers need to actively "restore the balance" and understand the meaning and emotional aspects of work for employees to create a more energised and fulfilled workforce [4]. Further studies reveal that organisations must attempt to actively engage with employees, which is the link to the triple bottom-line [5, 6]. Engaged employees aid the organisation to reach its mission, execute on its strategic goals and attain significant business results [5]. Whilst it is important to ensure that employees are adequately equipped to perform remotely, managers need to continuously engage and attain good rapport with their teams as this acts as a mediator to enhance behaviour, intention and attitude of employees, resulting in better work performance [4].

Remote Working and Commitment in Internal Auditing

Virtual arrangements amongst team members has been suggested to affect relationships and attitude of employees towards their organisations [6]. Under such a working environment, traditional performance measurements are not effective in motivating and engaging employees to commit further in their work, hence employers are looking at new ways to manage their employees [6]. Employee commitment is impacted by the way an employee feels about his/her job [6], and an engaged employee is an individual that is committed to his/her work and workplace [1]. Engagement increases when employees spend time both at an office workspace and through working remotely [1]. This blend of a hybrid working arrangement is posited to yield higher levels of engagement and hence commitment [1].

Commitment in a remote working environment is also influenced by an employee's level of concentration and focus, how distraction at the office workspace is greater than working from home. A home working environment is likely more constructive as it avoids "office talks" allowing for employees' greater focus on their work deliverables [7].

Employee Development and Effect on Productivity

Due to the pandemic, e-training platforms conducted thus far have given employees the desire to learn new subjects to aid in their development [8]. Organisations are buying more online training courses as opposed to previous in-house trainings [8]. Companies are benefiting with virtual training by saving on travel costs but are also expanding on the platforms of knowledge as courses offered are not restricted to specific locations. Whilst these are seen as positive actions from organisations in terms of investing and developing their employees, more is required to balance the increased online screen fatigue syndrome [8]. In another study, researchers used the components of emotional intelligence to determine the impact it has on career success and human resource development [9]. Their results showed that emotional intelligence does help workers to achieve success in the workplace and that more focus must be paid to developing employee's emotional intelligence at work. It can be concluded that emotional intelligence successfully develops an employee through their activities and levels of career development. Whilst initially intellectual abilities may advance career development, in the long term emotional intelligence will contribute significantly to one's career advancement. Hence, it is recommended that individuals pay attention to a particular skill for future success and improve their emotional intelligence through emotional training.

However, another study posits [10] that partial remote audit can be conducted where auditors are on-site when they need to be. This is similar to a hybrid model where employees come into the office to work on-site with clients. They also mention that the use of a modern technological auditing tool will aid in advancing the way audits are done, improving their assurance and advisory services, and reducing costs of the audit process as reports are electronically set up. Furthermore, auditing tools increase productivity, and saves time and effort in producing audit programs which in turn increase the speed and efficiencies of the audit process [10].

The Future of Communication through Emotional Agility

Online communication over extended periods of time can become tiresome and may lead to distractions. Interactions on virtual communities arise where employees, employers and clients can engage and interact but they may lose interest or commitment to the relationship over time [11]. Results revealed that social interaction and group connections have a significant effect on participation and that member-to-member interaction is encouraged [11]. It is recommended that in order to motivate employees to interact socially, employers must consider a relationship-retaining strategy. Online interaction and social interconnectedness are essential for employees to maintain good working relationships even in the virtual community, and it is suggested that current topics of interest can be presented to employees to discuss in the virtual space.

Another study also concurs by stating that communication efficiency through the use of online platforms can be tedious as more instructions are needed to clearly and effectively communicate expectations and confirm understanding. These authors further argue that while online communication promotes divergent thinking, convergent thinking and reaching consensus is more effectively achieved in face-to-face engagements. Furthermore, they explain that physical communication promotes quicker information flow and encourages greater participation [12].

Tools to Develop Employees During Remote Working

Developing employees requires not only providing the opportunities for effective training facilities during remote working but extra effort is needed from leaders to support and guide their teams to achieve successful growth. This does not just mean growth towards a specific position within the organisation but also includes self-development. Emotional intelligence awareness is increasingly becoming recognised as an integral part of one's leadership [13]. Workplaces previously would impede emotions as the latter were never considered as part of the workplace phenomenon. However, another study [13] evaluated how emotions can impact and be managed in order to improve outcomes in the work environment. Their research studied five constructs of emotional intelligence in the workspace, namely, "self-awareness, self-regulation, internal motivation, empathy, social skills" [13]. It revealed how leaders can become more efficient and effective not only through the demonstrated personality and cognition traits, but also to lead by gaining a deeper understanding of behaviour in order to develop employees and achieve optimum performance.

In addition, effective leaders should employ emotional agility that addresses emotions in a mindful and productive way [13]. Therefore, an effective work environment must be open to emotional intelligence as it offers awareness on appropriate or inappropriate behaviours enabling effective communication engagement, which in essence enhances personal development.

Employee Well-Being During Remote Working

An employee's well-being directly impacts each of the three constructs of engagement, commitment and development as it is the foundation on which all human beings function. In terms of emotional stability and employee well-being during the pandemic, leaders will be looked up to and will have to guide each and every employee on emotional stability and how to overcome their emotional stresses [14].

Well-being includes supporting employees to take care of their families. This is corroborated by a study showing that employees experience greater job satisfaction as work-family conflict is reduced, telecommuting increases and autonomy is enhanced through remote working [15].

The aim of this chapter was to reflect on how necessary it is for leaders in business today to be more emotionally intelligent in order to take their organisations to greater heights. An additional study [16] reveals that an individual's emotional intelligence and self-concept are the essential aspects of one's mental well-being. They looked at the changing dynamics of the business world and the extent of disruptive events such as the COVID-19 pandemic, Industry 4.0[a] and the emergence of new technologies. They postulate the essential significance of the mental well-being of humans during a disruptive work environment.

---

[a] According to the World Economic Forum, Industry 4.0 is a digital revolution where technologies between the digital, physical and biological spheres are becoming more integrated and comprehensive.

Emotional intelligence is considered as the capacity to accurately understand one's emotions, to recognise the messages that emotions transmit, and to self-control one's emotions [16]. This can be construed to mean adapting oneself in terms of understanding their emotions and reactions to the situation [16]. An organisation's leader should see themselves as guiding and directing employees on how to be more resilient. According to the authors, organisations are changing in a manner today called a "new norm", such that it is not only the organisation itself that needs to see how they do business but business leaders themselves as well [16]. As a result, mental and emotional intelligence play a critical role in a disruptive environment [16]. People who have better control over their feelings and emotions are better able to make decisions quickly, are empathic to others' feelings, are self-directed and can better manage problems [16]. Remote working will be a new norm post-pandemic and those who understand their remote working employees by continuously engaging with them, dealing with conflict management amongst their team members, and developing leader-team member relationships can emerge as an effective leader [16]. They further elaborate that in as much as radical changes are occurring, those with good mental and emotional capabilities will support critical thinking needed to take strategic actions beyond the disruptive business environment. It is crucial to have an understanding of the factors that affect employee well-being during remote working, as well as the way employees feel, which affect their productivity and ultimately deplete human capital investment in the organisation.

Organisational and Employee Agility

In order to better grasp the psychological effects of human traits and choices during the COVID-19 pandemic [17], a study reviewed three adaptive traits, namely, grit, resilience, and emotional agility to understand how those who are adaptive to changes are more likely to survive than those that who are static. It would be important to understand from internal audit's management what behavioural changes were noted and how they were dealt with. It was revealed that grit sustains a powerful disciplined motivation to achieve one's goals, resilience allows one to recover quickly from difficult circumstances, and emotional agility is a self-managed approach to lessen stress, approach problems adaptively and continuously refine performance. The traits highlighted in this study are deemed necessary to equip the next generation to become more capable of adapting to any changes. This review of extant literature highlights the dire need for organisations and individuals to become more agile and flexible in order to survive the world in the future.

Theoretical Frameworks

Two conceptual frameworks were used to critique the impact each construct has on the concepts of the models and frameworks, namely Freeman's stakeholder theory (1984) and Penrose's resource-based view of the firm (1959). Freeman's stakeholder theory addresses how the factors of internal audit's communication, commitment, and development impact all stakeholders [20,21]. The impact of internal audit's employee engagement, commitment, and development during remote working has been assessed against these services.

Penrose's resource-based view of the firm (1959) adequately conceptualises the internal factors to consider for the internal auditing work environment and proves to be valid in analysing how employee engagement, commitment, and development will affect the unit's effectiveness [22]. The advantage of using this model is its focus on looking at past experiences of employee engagement, commitment, and development, which are used to understand what the future expectations could be based on the purpose of the internal audit function.

Methodology

The Design of the Study

To achieve the research objectives, this study followed a qualitative research approach. To gather the research data, the study comprised two important parts, a comprehensive literature review and fieldwork. An exploratory research design, consisting of semi-structured interview questions as the research instrument, was chosen for this study. The reason for using an exploratory research design is that very little knowledge is available on the implication of remote working in the internal auditing environment. Exploratory studies provide key information where little data exist and can be useful in understanding the magnitude of a problem or phenomenon. This type of research design aims to explain ambiguous circumstances or uncover potential business opportunities. Hence the aim of this research was to understand the impact of remote working on employee engagement, commitment, and development through interviews.

Sampling Strategy and Primary Data Collection Method

The purpose of the qualitative method is to collect data from credible resources that would produce significant knowledge to inform the research objectives. Detailed information is provided for readers to understand the procedures undertaken and to make their own judgement of the quality of information provided in the study [18]. Ethical standards were applied throughout as all required permissions were obtained through each step of the research process.

The purposive sampling strategy was used, which is a non-probability technique where judgement has been used to select the individuals that make up the sample [19]. The characteristics of the group of participants selected provided in-depth information about the employees' agility during remote working. The purposive sampling technique has been applied to the participants chosen to reflect the diversity of the IAU.

The sample size selected was 10 senior managers at the IAU in the eThekwini Municipality. This sampling strategy was most convenient as it allowed this specific group to be targeted. Based on this group's particular characteristics, they would be aware of emotional and behavioural changes in their employees before and during the pandemic as they have direct contact and communication with them. The employees of the IAU also report directly to the senior managers on administrative issues, productivity, and training and career development. The senior managers have a responsibility to both lead and manage their teams to understand their behaviours, needs and wants and have the capacity to understand what would be most suitable for their teams.

The sampling was specifically focused on senior management as they represent the staff they lead and are expected to manage emotional agility in the IAU work environment for the employees. The interviewees for the qualitative research were chosen based on their seniority and agility experience in the IAU. Online interviews were conducted with Executive and Senior managers within the IAU. This particular group of individuals would have in-depth knowledge of the remote working conditions of their employees and are in senior management positions to evaluate employee agility. This group manages communication, development and ensure that commitment is maintained in the unit. At management level, this group of individuals are expected to provide recommendations to improve communication, development, and commitment amongst their teams. They are also expected to take note of the well-being of their employees.

Primary Data Analysis Method

The primary data analysis technique used for this study was thematic. A theme is a broad category combining many codes that appear to be interrelated to each other and indicates a concept or idea that links to the research question of the study. The qualitative information obtained from the interviews were thematically coded and analysed. Coding entails a process of labelling data using a code that summarises the meaning of the data [19]. The advantage of using a thematic analysis is that it offers a systematic, orderly approach to analysing data in a logical manner. The transcripts retrieved electronically were cleaned and the information and viewpoints from each participant were carefully analysed. The cleaning of the transcripts involved a process of removing duplicated words or repeated expressions that were captured and transcribed automatically by the electronic recording process during the online interviews. In this study the audio recordings were replayed to ensure that information transcribed was not misinterpreted. Subsequently, key and minimised bias viewpoints were extracted from each participant. This information was further condensed into specific themes and categorised into positive and negative responses.

Ethical Considerations

Ethical considerations have been made in the preliminary, planning, implementation and concluding stages of the research study. An ethical clearance and a gatekeeper permission letter were obtained. Consent from participants had been obtained before interviews and were recorded. The privacy of participants' details was preserved by numbering each participant in order to ensure anonymity. All information collected and recorded have been kept securely in electronic files. A brief induction was provided to the participants to assure them of the confidentiality of the research and to ensure authenticity in their responses. A high level of confidentially was maintained while participants expressed their challenges on the remote working operations of their organisation. Forms of bias such as influencing comments, change of tone or any non-verbal behaviour to impose on interviewee responses have been avoided. The researcher's objectivity was maintained throughout the interview process, analysing and reporting of data to avoid any bias conclusions [19]. All primary data-related matters were managed with ethical integrity.

Analysis and Discussion of the Findings

The data collected from the semi-structured qualitative research interview questions were used to determine how the factors of emotional agility affected the IAU's productivity during remote working. Thematic analysis had been used to derive the set of findings among the three constructs of employee engagement, commitment levels, and development. Quotes from the participants were used to validate responses to questions posed in the interview. Specific details of these themes and participant responses follow.

a) *Comfort of your home*

It was noted that individuals were more comfortable at home during remote working and, as a result, there was more participation and engagement. "Comfort at home" was mentioned by five participants. It became more convenient for them to communicate using the various forms of technology.

b) *Effective communication*

Three participants mentioned that communication also became quick and easy, and people were flexible and were available on extended hours of the day. People were more expressive and participation in online meetings increased. One response was that due to the absence of physical presence in meetings, "people would speak up more." Another participant added that apart from the evidence of saving on travelling time and costs, employees found it easier to communicate remotely as being office-based meant that sometimes individuals would wait for others to arrive for a meeting.

c) *Lack of stimulation*

The main concern that emerged from five out of the ten individuals in terms of the negative perspective of communication was that there was lack of stimulation, and absence of interaction and body language when remotely working. Two participants mentioned that more effort was needed to contact a person, to the extent that it would take up more time to get a message through. An individual mentioned that "Human interaction was missing on a digital space," as online calls do not provide the full social compliment. It was noted that some internal auditors had become quiet during remote working and participated less during online meetings.

d) *Commitment doubled*

There were six out of ten responses that revealed commitment had been shown from employees during remote working. Comments such as "commitment doubled", "commitment was high", or "my team showed full commitment" were received. A participant noted that some colleagues were asking to also go to the office because they understood that even though they were working remotely, they did not want remote working to be the downfall of their projects. This participant also mentioned that auditors were willing to go on-site and meet with clients. Three participants noted that employees were more available even if calls were made to them after the normal hours of work (*i.e.*, from 8 am to 5 pm).

e) *Flexibility encouraged output of work*

The results show that three out of ten participants made mention of the fact that due to the flexible working hours, people can deliver in the best time that suits them. One participant mentioned that "they are seeing to their personal errands so in return they deliver the work even if they have to work at night."

f) *Cost savings*

Five participants mentioned that online trainings were free which allowed them to develop themselves. On the other hand, two participants mentioned that budget constraints for training courses was seen as a limitation during the remote working period. As a result, suppliers reduced the cost over time.

g) *Personal growth development*

Five out of the ten participants stated that online training enhanced development and skills of internal auditors during remote working due to the following factors: the use of technology offered courses to a wider group of individuals as there was no limitation to have training in certain locations; and personal growth of employees increased as they took to the free online training offered by many external stakeholders and professional bodies. Overall, the results showed that skills and development of employees were ongoing and, in certain instances, grew.

h) *Human disconnection*

Four participants noted that there was a sense of disconnection as no contact training was available. It was mentioned that this would impact young graduates' development in the long term as they would not be exposed to the presence of facilitators, hindering the completeness of the learning process. Another participant added on by saying that virtual training was not as effective as face-to-face training as body language and the transfer of practical skills are absent on the virtual platform.

i) *Acknowledgement of work*

The main theme that emanated from seven participants on this question was that acknowledgment of employee performance would enhance commitment. Participant 1 listed tacit rewards such as "allowing people time off on a Friday afternoon, or recognising they just travelled and need time on Monday to attend to family or kids." Valuing a person's effort and acknowledging them in an open platform by having workshops was recommended by another participant. Show appreciation, saying "Thank you" and "Well done", recognising when good work is done, providing encouragement, finding innovative ways of keeping people motivated, were other prominent responses. These participants concurred that when individuals are productive, that reflects their commitment.

j) *Connection and socialisation*

Four participants mentioned that teamwork should be encouraged during this time to show support for each other. Connection and communication are important during this time.

Participant 10 explained how a company had introduced a social online, where staff were asked to send pictures of themselves working remotely with families, or videos of activities they were busy with during this time. In doing this the organisation showed that they cared about their employees' well-being and their families. This was seen as a great initiative to show a fun side to work.

Participant 9 explained that Heritage Day celebrations and birthdays that used to be held by the unit would encourage employees. Also, recognition of people who lost families. This participant mentioned that positive feedback from clients is recognition of the good work being carried out by the team.

k) *Growth and study support*

The outcome of results for this question varied amongst each senior manager whilst the most prominent theme was to encourage and motivate staff to grow and study. This was stated by six of the ten participants. It was noted that it is not only about developing just the individual but also the organisation, and that time must be allocated for learning. Participant 1 stated that 'as a manager' one needs to communicate with people about where they see themselves in their careers. Another participant mentioned that the IAU needed to encourage and motivate auditors for them to upskill, develop and study.

l) *Deep discussions*

Three participants mentioned that employees need one-on-one discussions and leaders must invest time in deep discussion and conversation to understand the challenges and opportunities in people. A participant stated that a leader really needs to push themselves to develop their teams, and as a manager one needs to create that platform for employees to develop. This participant was assertive by saying that "I can't be pushing them, I need them to add value, and study and really research, then every year becomes a year of new discoveries."

m) *Knowledge*

Knowledge sharing and the growth of knowledge was combined as a common theme from three participants. A participant recommended that the unit could invite a guest speaker to talk about any relevant and latest audit topic in workshop sessions. Participant 2 highlighted that continuous development is essential based on the requirements of their professional registrations. Professional bodies offer online courses that can be shared with the teams. Participant 6 proposed that individuals who attended training with professional bodies could provide feedback and re-present the skill or concept taught to the rest of the teams.

Participant 3 revealed that in terms of self-development, there was more time available in the day for people to research more. The advice was to take advantage of the time available and engage more with content, learn and research more. In summary, learning platforms have expanded and broadened and "short-courses" are offered now, which means that an individual's workplace skills plan can be achieved.

n) *Empathy and compassion*

Three of the ten participants noted that employees have most definitely changed in behaviour; some are more compassionate and empathetic, and others have become more reserved. The participants observed that employees understood that we all have been affected by this pandemic, hence under the circumstances of working, it was important to have a work-life balance. People are realising that there is much more room for growth as remote working has given people time to reflect. A participant stated that encouragement through "building relationships and connections", by giving people calls not about work but about their own well-being, would show their worth and value.

o) *Maturity and trust*

Five of the ten participants noted that remote working gave way to building more trust with employees who in turn also showed maturity by delivering their work. The first participant mentioned that maturity is evident in employees as people are taking on more responsibility and accountability for their actions. A participant highlights that "with freedom comes responsibility", as there is no longer a systematic way of operating: now the responsibility is on the individual to manage him/herself. Remote working has given leaders the opportunity to realise that the more you trust people the more they react, and the more commitment is received.

Participant 9 observed that typically when remotely working, there is a tendency to not trust staff and to performance manage them. However, staff should be communicated with not for micromanaging purposes, but to check in on them once a week to create a little openness and transparency. It was acknowledged that staff are also parents and have family commitments but, in the team, with some level of trust it smoothens out potential conflicts and generates openness. This in turn helps employees with their well-being.

p) *Work-life balance*

Three participants mentioned that individuals must have a balance between work and family. Participant 2 mentioned that remote working encouraged a "work-life balance" and improved their mental well-being as individuals in a way that enables them to allocate time to deal with whatever personal matters they need to do and then be able to be present themselves fully when they are doing work, which results in the reduction of errors. From this perspective it is as if they are doing what they know they ought to do, but without having to ask, which shifts their behaviour towards a more confident way of living. Another participant added that quality time could be spent with family by helping with the children's homework during the day and be able to produce work till late at night.

The 7th participant stated that in terms of wellness of employees, staff had the flexibility to lead a less stressful lifestyle, with less traffic congestion and more family time, and it was fruitful to do other things which contributed to work-life balance. It was further mentioned that remote working had made it flexible for employees to do their own chores, which in a way uplifted their wellness point of view; however, they still had to be committed to delivering their work.

q) *Emotional wellness*

Three participants took note that employees had experienced personal issues over the pandemic and were referred to the City's wellness clinic to assist and support them. They acknowledged that when employees are not performing well, they need further consultation and can be referred to the municipality's wellness clinic.

To be excellent in and to uphold its services, the IAU's biggest asset is its human capital, which was the main focus in this study. The aim of this research was to understand the extent of agility in employees during remote working by looking at how they communicated with each other, their levels of commitment to work and the organisation, and the development of their skills. It must be observed that this study was a cross-sectional review, which gave way to remarks and suggestions that emanated from the current point in time of the COVID-19 pandemic. However, the key focus of this study was to assess how employees of internal auditing adapted to the circumstances of remote working and to understand if this work environment setup was beneficial or not for the unit to provide its professional mandate in the long term.

Overall, the results reveal that engagement, commitment, and development of internal auditors was well during remote working and in some instances improved with technology. This means that agility and adaptability were evident in all three constructs. As with any process and operational changes, there are teething problems. These have been pointed out by various participants and need further improvement. One major glaring concern is that employees are needing social interaction and physical human presence during this time.

The agility of employees to adapt to communication, commitment and training, and development during remote working was mostly received in the affirmative. There were reflections on individuals' internal perceptions such as "willpower" in making online training a success. Participants in certain instances also reflected on how productivity was evident, which showed ability by employees to adapt in showing commitment during remote working. The various platforms used for communication gave all participants confidence in the ongoing engagements with employees and this reflected full adaptability.

As explained in the literature review, the "connection" with individuals was necessary during remote working and employers need to restore the balance to create and energise an active workforce [4]. There were positive viewpoints from participants in terms of the extent of courses offered to a larger group which gave employees the opportunities to learn more during remote working, corroborated by [8].

However, the literature [8] supports the fact that employees do feel tired and have "fatigue" when doing online training, which has also been stressed upon by participants. The distractions experienced at home during training sessions [7] show that this is true; however, distractions are also experienced in face-to-face or office training. This study [7] also observed that employees have a high job satisfaction and in return performance is increased. The senior management participants have noted the same outcome in that remote working does not only increase employee morale but also productivity.

There will be a sense of mistrust in employees when remotely working due to the lack of physical presence [4], but as one participant mentioned, it requires building open and transparent relationships with employees to "smoothen out trust", thereby uplifting their well-being and commitment. A participant who mentioned that employers need to give employees the opportunity to have a work-life balance is also supported by extant literature [4].

A comment received by one participant mentioned that the office was not conducive in terms of health and safety risks due to poor building conditions and that working from home made employees feel safe. This is also endorsed by the research study [3] that showed low emotional agility existed at an unsafe work environment as it was more challenging and stressful.

Communication channels need to be open [5]. Additionally, reverting to the traditional ways of operating would not be effective in motivating and enhancing commitment from employees to work [6]. A participant also contributes to this by stating that it would not be conducive as the extra hours of operating would not be suitable in the full-time office setup.

Participant responses in terms of the hybrid model being the best approach is also iterated in the literature [1], which explains that employee engagements increase when they spend time both at the office and remotely. Reference is made to the study [9] that reflected that grooming an employee's emotional intelligence builds them to become more resilient and promotes future vitality. This directly matches with some participants' viewpoints on investing more time in employees to motivate them to study and groom them to manage their time optimally. This illustrates that both the theory and participants' feedback correspond to say career growth and learning are self-made and require introspection.

The literature and data analysis both agree that adapting to remote working leads to both positive and negative outcomes. Participants affirmed that an automated auditing system will promote their services and will ensure successful adoption to the new way of working and researchers agreed that this was a fundamental tool to have. The hybrid model was accepted by both the overall literature review and the participants of this study as the best approach to operating internal audit services.

With reference to Freeman's stakeholder theory, in terms of development, participants mentioned that their external training providers were relied upon to provide online training courses. Some of these training providers had moved to online training with agility, yet others had teething problems initially but had later provided training with larger and a wider range of courses being made available. If such training services were not provided timeously or were not made available online, auditors' skills and development would have been hindered. This would have created a ripple effect on their services and output to clients in the local government municipality. In terms of communication and commitment, some participants mentioned how clients were impacted as some had to spend a lot of time scanning documents for internal auditing requests. Other clients did not easily adapt to online communication and needed auditors to come on-site. This meant that internal auditors had to make themselves available to meet the client's needs. The recommendation, as mentioned by a few participants, was to obtain an automated auditing system. This would positively improve the impact and outcome of communication, commitment, and development of the Internal Audit team amongst all stakeholders.

As per the Penrose's resource-based view model, and with reference to the viewpoint from the participants, it was evident that all processes from the model could be applied. It was essential to making every audit team's output a success. Process one requires an effective team to have material resources and human resources. The internal auditors were provided with 3G cards, data, access to email, MS Teams, and the internet. In process two, the teams' past experience of operating in an office-based environment and the current remote working environment were assessed. The use of technological resources together with the combined efforts of internal audit staff during remote working gave way to "subjective productive opportunities", which led to productive services. This was displayed in steps 3 and 4 of the model. The senior managers also saw growth and maturity within individuals during the time of remote working, and employees were exposed to many diverse platforms of communication as well as to training platforms of online seminars and webinars. These factors contributed to the growth and development of employees during remote working. The senior managers in this study provided feedback on the "rate of growth" and "mode of growth" within their teams. The outcome was that online training broadened their knowledge base. During this time participants noted how employees self-reflected and realised the time available during remote working could be used as an opportunity to grow and self-develop. The model showed how the "development of underutilised productive services" could be an outcome of remote working, but through the agility of auditing teams, growth and development was still encouraged. This was reflected in processes 5, 6 and 7 in the model.

The learning resources and the rate of growth will be evidenced through the way internal audit deploys resources such as provision of services and solutions to clients that are innovative and efficient (step 8). The direction of the IAU in its current and diverse "new norm" circumstance that it finds itself in, together with its current resources that are continuously growing and developing in skills and knowledge, will ultimately lead to the unit's effectiveness and a "competitive advantage" in utilising its resources effectively. The current sequence of events through remote working has actually proven to lead the audit teams in a successful manner provided that continuous training and development and technological support are provided to employees during remote working. The Penrose resource-based view model thus addresses how the factors of communication, commitment, and development impact the productivity of internal auditors as a team during remote working that will guide them to achieving their units' objectives and goals.

It is crucial for organisations to delve into the benefits of remote working, because as recommended in a particular study [7], when morale improves and is upheld, employers will gain great benefits from excellent working employees. This in turn will translate to better performance and productivity outputs as displayed in Penrose's resource-based view, and would lead to greater organisational performance satisfying the needs of various stakeholders referred to in Freeman's stakeholder theory. Hence the objective of this study has been attained in that organisations who invest in understanding emotional agility in employees positively influences productivity for internal auditors while working remotely.

Conclusions and Recommendations

The objective of the research was to answer one underlying question: "What is the extent of emotional agility such as employee engagement, commitment, and development that influences productivity of internal auditors while working remotely?" To achieve this, ten interviews with the IAU senior management were conducted to provide insights in which the participants articulated their agile transitioning experiences with employees.

The most significant discovery in this study is that emotional agility cannot improve by moving back to the office full-time as the successes and benefits of working remotely exceed office-based productivity. Employers need to carefully examine creating an environment that is flexible to accommodate all types of employees, especially considering their well-being from a holistic point of view, and work on emotional and behavioural changes where necessary. Investment in people leads to investment in organisational growth.

The research study has found that the limitations of traditional culture and methods had a cascading effect on the profession, hindering the potential of the IAU to be agile and enhance employee engagement, commitment, and development during remote working. Some recommendations proposed address these traditional setbacks, to improve the IAU morale in a remote working setup to enable the unit to pivot during this transition. These tools are provided to show how the benefits of the transition from office based to remote working are enough to justify why it was important for the IAU to overcome any challenges faced during its adoption.

Recommendations include the following:

i) *The hybrid approach*

The Internal Audit function within the administration of the City should consider formalising a hybrid approach with clear formal ground rules in terms of productivity and operational requirements for internal auditors. Creating a hybrid auditing framework with clear computations and control mechanisms will give other stakeholders within the municipality the reasons and justifications of the transition.

ii) *Integrated working*

One major challenge that was evident is that internal auditors tend to be more reserved, and management has found that even when communicating, they are limited to only communication within their teams, resulting in silo output. A platform to enhance integration amongst teams is needed. This would increase productivity and quality of services provided by the team [10].

iii) *Socialisation*

Human interaction and body language was found to be lacking significantly. The leadership of the IAU need to address the issues of "disconnection." Employers are encouraged to keep employees engaged during remote working and keep their minds active to promote an energised and active workforce [5]. Although organisations are benefitting by saving on catering, travel and accommodation costs, for online training more is required to reduce the increased online screen fatigue syndrome [8]. Participants recommended that virtual interactions through 3D headsets or having online social gatherings would benefit the well-being of the team. The hybrid model allows for more interaction both online and at the office.

iv) *Knowledge sharing*

In terms of continuous development, enabling employees to be engaged in learning, training and development interventions on what trainees themselves have been taught would promote growth for everyone to grow at a faster rate. Professional articles on specific and relevant topics can be distributed and shared amongst teams.

v) *Building trust*

For employees who had shown no commitment even before the pandemic [1], the best approach is probably to ask the employee how s/he feels about the job, and to consult him/her further. Invest time in employees by grooming them to manage themselves. Allow them to reflect on their own self-development. Supporting these employees would mean to encourage better relationships [12]. Both employers and employees must seek to rebuild the culture of trust.

vi) *Audit software tool*

An automated audit system would increase the speed and efficiency of audit services provided [10]. The audit team would be able to expand and increase the provision of assurance and consulting services.

Further studies should include all employees in the internal audit function rather than a sample of senior audit managers. This approach can provide quantitative feedback on how employees have been affected directly. Quantitative and qualitative studies through surveys and interviews can also be conducted on other internal audit municipal functions in other provinces in order to assess emotional agility of internal auditors across the country at large.

References

[1] Lee, AM (2018). An exploratory case study of how remote employees experience workplace engagement. *Walden Dissertations and Doctoral Studies.* https://scholarworks.waldenu.edu/dissertations/5569/.

[2] Kamilah, H & Hanifah (2021). Construction and validation of emotional agility measurement tools: measuring one's emotional agility. *JPPP — Jurnal Penelitian dan Pengukuran Psikologi*, **10**(1), 65–72.

[3] Mishra, I & Panwar, DN (2020). Emotional agility on working employees under Indian conditions. *The International Journal of Indian Psychology*, **8**(2), 1367–1375.

[4] Cartwright, S & Holmes, N (2006). The meaning of work: the challenge of regaining employee engagement and reducing cynicism. *Human Resource Management Review*, **16**(2), 199–208.

[5] Chanana, N & Sangeeta (2020). Employee engagement practices during COVID-19 lockdown. *Journal of Public Affairs*, **21**(4), e2508. DOI:10.1002/pa.2508

[6] Howell, DC (2018). Virtual employee engagement identifying best practices for engaging a remote workforce (Masters Dissertation). *Pepperdine University*. https://www.proquest.com/openview/3b18be5a194bb5be780fde4940f184e2/1?pq-origsite=gscholar&cbl=18750.

[7] Lassiter, V (2020). The differences in job satisfaction, engagement, and dedication between full-time remote and non-remote employees (Doctorate Thesis). *Trevecca Nazarene University*. https://www.proquest.com/openview/658e4f38ed66a17cbd8d2c6166adf758/1?pq-origsite=gscholar&cbl=18750&diss=y.

[8] Mikołajczyk, K (2021). Changes in the approach to employee development in organisations as a result of the COVID-19 pandemic. *European Journal of Training and Development*, **46**(5–6), 544–562.

[9] Chagelishvili, A (2021). The contribution of emotional intelligence to human resource development and career success: a review. *European Journal of Economics and Business Studies*, 7(2), 49–59.

[10] Serag, AAEM & Daoud, MM (2021). Remote auditing: an alternative approach to face the internal audit challenges during the COVID-19 pandemic. *The Accounting Thought Journal*, **25**(2), 228–259.

[11] Shih-Tse Wang, E, Shui-Lien Chen, L & Tsai, BK (2012). Investigating member commitment to virtual communities using an integrated perspective. *Internet Research*, **22**(2), 199–210.

[12] Teeter, RA & Vasarhelyi, MA (2010). Remote audit: a review of audit enhancing information and communication technology literature. *SSRN*. https://dx.doi.org/10.2139/ssrn.2488732.

[13] Cavaness, K, Picchioni, A & Fleshman, JW (2020). Linking emotional intelligence to successful health care leadership: the big five model of personality. *Clinics in Colon and Rectal Surgery*, **33**(4), 195–203.

[14] Dirani, KM, Abadi, M, Alizadeh, A, Barhate, B, Garza, RC, Gunasekara, N & Majzun, Z (2020). Leadership competencies and the essential role of human resource development in times of crisis: a response to COVID-19 pandemic. *Human Resource Development International*, **23**(4), 380–394.

[15] Schall, MA (2019). The relationship between remote work and job satisfaction: The mediating roles of perceived autonomy, work-family conflict, and telecommuting

intensity (Masters Thesis). *San Jose State University.* https://scholarworks.sjsu.edu/etd_theses/5017/.

[16] Vaidya, RW, Prasad, K & Mangipudi, MR (2020). Mental and emotional competencies of leader's dealing with disruptive business environment — a conceptual review. *International Journal of Management,* **11**(5), 366–375.

[17] Suppawittayaa, P, Busarakulb, T, Wangwongwirojc, T & Yasrid, P (2021). Psychological adaptation after the COVID-19 pandemic through the lens of evolutionary biology. *Systematic Reviews in Pharmacy,* **12**(3), 788–794.

[18] Creswell, JW & Creswell, JD (2018). *Research Design: Qualitative, Quantitative, and Mixed Methods Approaches* (5th ed.). SAGE.

[19] Saunders, M, Lewis, P & Thornhill, A (2019). *Research Methods for Business Students* (8th ed.). Pearson Education.

[20] Gomes, RC (2006). Stakeholder management in the local government decision-making area: evidences from a triangulation study with the English local government. *Brazilian Administration Review,* **3**(1), 46–63.

[21] Pajunen, K (2010). A "black box" of stakeholder thinking. *Journal of Business Ethics,* **96**(S1), 27–32.

[22] Kor, YY & Mahoney, JT (2002). Penrose's resource-based approach: the process and product of research creativity. *Journal of Management Studies,* **37**, 109–139.

Chapter

9

The Lessons of Past Pandemics

By AC Grayling

Summary

The dramatic demographic and scientific changes that have occurred in the world over the last 70 years in some key respects limit the value of comparisons between COVID-19 and previous major pandemics. Yet some lessons remain from past experience; both the comparisons and differences between the circumstances in which COVID-19 occurred and those of past pandemics tell us much about what is needed for confronting the increasing threat of future pandemic diseases.

It should come as no surprise that the answer to the question, 'What can we learn from previous major pandemics in history?', is in *some* respects: 'rather little'. The chief reason is that the remarkable growth in scientific knowledge and capability since the mid-20th century has made responding to pandemic disease greatly more effective, especially in epidemiology, vaccination development, clinical practice, and countermeasures including public information, control of population movement at critical periods, and the ability to identify and address sources of disease outbreak.

But history is never entirely without lessons. Epidemics and pandemics litter the human record; in the Common Era (the last two thousand years) there has been a number of notable examples — the Plague of Justinian (541–43), the Black Death (1347–51), repeated cholera pandemics in the 19th century, the Spanish Flu (1918–19), to say nothing of more localised outbreaks of plague (such as those in Venice in 1575 and London in 1665–66). And the 21st century has already seen SARS-CoV (2002–03), Swine Flu (2009–10), MERS-CoV (2015–continuing), and COVID-19 (SARS-CoV-2, 2019–continuing).

Consider what difference current techniques in these respects would have made to the Black Death. That outbreak of bubonic plague, caused by the *Yersinia pestis* bacterium carried by black rats (*Rattus rattus*) and their fleas, body lice and bedbugs, and spread secondarily in aerosols causing pneumonic plague, resulted in an estimated 75–200 million fatalities, in the case of Europe reducing the continent's population by 30–40%, though more than this in England and less in Poland. Had there been today's resources for responding to the Black Death, matters would have been far different. Epidemiological analysis would have caught its onset at an earlier stage, and measures would have been adopted to limit its spread, treat its victims, eradicate its carriers, and immunise populations against it. Yet it was not until the work of Waldemar Haffkine at the end of the 19th century that a plague vaccine was developed; its vigorous use in India in the first quarter of the 20th century is estimated to have reduced plague mortality on the subcontinent by as much as 80%.

Epidemiology has been a key factor in the disjunction between past pandemic experience and now. Famously, physician John Snow's removal of the handle of a water pump in London's Soho district in 1854 helped to curtail that city's part in the repeated global cholera pandemics of the 19th century, a measure he took after tracing the incidence of the disease across the pump's local neighbourhoods. Although epidemiology can be said to have begun with Hippocrates, it is Snow who is accounted the 'father' of the science as a result. Coupled with improvements in both public and personal hygiene — for just one example: the wearing of underpants by larger sections of society from the 18th century onwards is credited with improving public health significantly — such developments have together changed the circumstances in which epidemic and pandemic disease can be confronted.

But it is the remarkable advances in the biological, biochemical and medical sciences that immeasurably widen the gulf between the past and present. Consider how much less severe the effects of the 1918–19 'Spanish' influenza epidemic would have been if the developments in virology and vaccine technology had preceded the outbreak. (The first Influenza A vaccine was licensed in 1945 after research and development began in the 1930s). Subsequently the revolution in biological science wrought by genetics has proved to be the key precursor to the miraculous-seeming speed with which vaccines were developed in response to COVID-19's outbreak. The lessons learned in virology and immunology, coupled to epidemiological analysis potentiated by artificial intelligence and computing speeds, are game changing with respect to future communicable disease management.

After the Black Death, labour shortages improved the lot of survivors because they were in demand and their standard of living rose. Erosion of feudal practices accompanied the change. It is unsurprising that major changes should result from so drastic a shock to economic and social conditions such as then prevailed, but matters are different now. In today's global economy, in a world vastly more populous and various, it is reasonable to expect negative impacts to be more limited and transient. At time of writing, the economic sequelae of COVID-19 are still evolving, rendered more difficult to evaluate because of the Russian invasion of Ukraine and consequent disruption to grain and energy supplies. Nevertheless some consequences are indeed visible: inflation and supply chain problems are among the most salient. But deeper and more diversified economies, more flexible financial instruments available to governments and internationally operating institutions such as banks, and existing resources of capital of all kinds, make for a degree of resilience lacking in former times. This implies a relatively short-term effect from economic impacts (see Chapter 6). Along with scientific developments, this is a major difference between COVID-19 and past pandemics. Other changes — most significantly to social, educational and working-life practices — are less obvious in the early stages but possibly more significant in the longer term, and it is here that comparisons with earlier pandemics are more instructive.

The most noticeable comparison is that major communicable disease outbreaks (including the various recent SARS and MERS coronavirus episodes) have all been preceded by marked and relatively rapid increases in population, urbanisation and population mobility. In the key examples of the Black Death in the years around 1350 and the Spanish Flu in 1918–19, the immediately preceding periods were also beset by military conflicts involving the movements of large bodies of men in arms, adding to the increasing number of sailors and merchants already then travelling between Asia, the Near East and Europe.

In the century before the Black Death the world's population expanded, and the *Pax Mongolica* of the 13th and early 14th centuries fostered trade from China along the Silk Roads to the Near East and Europe. Population increase was promoted by decades of climate conditions favourable to agriculture.

People were drawn in ever larger numbers to cities, which became crowded. In this same period the khanates which had succeeded the great empire of Genghis Khan were declining, and the south-westernmost of them, the Ilkhanate, came into conflict with the Genoese merchant outpost of Caffa in Crimea. This conflict flared into open warfare in 1344. Contemporaneously, conditions both in the Ilkhanate and in Europe were affected by a change in weather patterns causing a repeated series of poor harvests. Thus a congeries of factors was preparing the ground for a disaster.

It is hypothesised that Mongolian troops originally acquired the plague during 13th-century conquests in south-western China and the foothills of the Himalayas, and that the vector of the disease — fleas from black rats transported not just by rats themselves but in the manes of horses and on the clothing and luggage of soldiers — accompanied them back to the steppes and both eastward and westward in the khanates, slowly at first. Plague was identified in China in the mid-1330s. But it was — so it is surmised — the conflict between the Ilkhanate and the Genoese of Caffa that triggered the spread of the Black Death out of Asia. As they besieged Caffa, more and more of the Mongolian troops succumbed to the disease, reaching the point where men were dying faster than they could be buried. Their Khan, Janibeg, decided on the expedient of catapulting the corpses of plague victims into Caffa. As the plague spread in the city so its terrified population sought to flee, a number of ships succeeding in crossing the Black Sea to Constantinople and then on to the Greek archipelago, Sicily and the Italian mainland.

Moving at an average rate of two to two and a half miles a day, the plague spread across Italy, over the Alps and along the Mediterranean coast to France and Spain, and thence into central, eastern and northern Europe. The mortality rate was high; in the bubonic form, 30–60%; in the pneumonic form, 90–95%; in the septicaemic form, 100%. Because the mortality rate was so high — higher by far than in the Justinian plague of 543 and the various outbreaks in the centuries following 1350 — it has been hypothesised that there was an additional factor, a double pandemic perhaps, with Ebola or anthrax involved, in multiple waves in some regions brought in from different directions.

The English army returning from its triumph at Crecy in 1348, and the vigorous wool trade continuing across the Channel, were major factors in spreading the plague into the British Isles, with devastating effect. People succumbed at twice the rate of the rest of Europe; entire villages were wiped out, crops left standing in the fields, London's population halved. Thinking that the plague was an English disease, the Scots assembled an invasion army at Selkirk to profit from the devastation south of Hadrian's Wall, only for it to be all but exterminated by the Black Death where it camped.

Significantly, the region of Europe with the lowest mortality was Poland, whose king Casimir III 'the Great' closed the borders and enforced strict quarantine on anyone with the disease, walling sufferers into their homes. The striking result was a population mortality of only 15%. Another example of strict quarantine was Milan, where success in limiting the effects was nearly as great.

The factors involved — increased population, increased urbanisation, increased mobility of people and not least of large military cohorts on the move — required only the introduction of *Yersinia pestis* bacteria into the mix for a 'perfect storm' to follow. Much the same might be said about the Spanish Flu epidemic of 1918–19. The virus targeted the 18–40 age group primarily, theorists now thinking that older-aged cohorts had acquired partial immunity from a similar virus in the latter part of the 19th century. The affected group was, of course, the military-age group; millions of men and hundreds of thousands of women in auxiliary and medical services were mobilised and moved across the globe — troops from south Asia to the Near East and Europe, troops from the United States to Europe, troops within Europe moving east, west and south as the war raged in Flanders, on the Russian border, in Italy, and elsewhere. Some theoreticians suggest that the H1N1 Spanish A influenza virus was brought to Europe from South Asia; another is that it was a mutation from a virus causing acute respiratory distress disease in a British army camp in Flanders in 1916. Most plausible is the suggestion that its source was a military training camp, Funston, in Kansas in the US, in which young men from farming communities in that state's Haskell County lived in close contact with pigs and chickens and had been infected by the virus leaping from them into the local human population.

Population and its mobility, now both vastly greater than in the Spanish Flu's conditions of opportunity in 1918, are such obvious factors in pandemic disease risk that they would be scarcely worth mentioning were it not that they identify one of the key lessons: the need for measures assiduously monitoring outbreaks and immediately and comprehensively stopping movement out of outbreak localities. Criticism of China's employment of this technique in the

COVID-19 crisis has several prompts, the chief being the economic impact of immobilising an entire city as was done in Shanghai and elsewhere. But the even greater cost of an uncontrolled pandemic is a persuasive rebuttal to that criticism.

The ability to mount swift early responses to threat is contingent on preparedness. A particular lesson to be wrung from past pandemics is that because they could neither be predicted nor, once raging, sufficiently controlled — ignorance of the vectors of disease typically subverted all control efforts apart from quarantine — it is pointless to accuse governments in 1350, 1850 or 1918 of failing to be prepared; but in 2020 this accusation could indeed be levelled, at some governments at least. Complacency, cost cutting, allowing supplies of such necessities as personal protective equipment to fall out of date, ignoring the advice of emergency planning committees, neglecting emergency training, underfunding broad-spectrum research that tries to anticipate where and in what manner major disease threats might appear, are culpable matters. Given that population densities and mobility continue to grow and with ever-increasing rapidity, demography alone ensures that pandemics will not only be inevitable but will likely increase in frequency. Therefore, preparedness is all: and it is fortunate that the appropriate science is available to ensure that we ('we': humanity) can be optimally prepared if the will — expressed, of course, in terms of funding — is available.

Some of the changes flowing from the COVID-19 pandemic are inevitable. One is the hastening of processes that were already in train. A prime example is the practice of office staff working more from home (see Chapter 8). With the advent of ubiquitous computing power in small devices, the need to be on site disappears for many kinds of occupations, most typically for office work and administration. The climate change pressure exerted by commuting had already begun to make some think that increased levels of working from home would be a useful contribution to addressing the climate emergency. 'Lockdown' demonstrated to millions the feasibility and advantages of doing so (and of course some of the disadvantages), with the result that in many workplaces there has been a shift to dividing time between working from home and attending the office. It is reasonable to expect that this trend will continue and likely increase, and in doing so will have further social and economic impacts. For a random example: if people are not travelling into the city so often, they will require more resources for shopping, leisure and amenity in local neighbourhoods, and correlatively some sectors of the economy — transport, and those businesses dependent on volumes of commuters passing their premises — will see revenues decline. Correlatively, business opportunities and revenues of existing local outlets will rise.

In past pandemics — those before the 19th century, certainly — most people already worked from home. Because they did so, the resources for subsistence tended to be home produced or available locally. Habits of daily life were not as dramatically altered as is now envisaged for a world where living and working in different localities has become the norm — in historical terms, a practice that began very recently indeed. From the viewpoints of disease spread, climate impact, lifestyle effects of commuting time and separation of work and non-work life experience, this recent shift appears unsustainable, and the pre-existing model might therefore reassert itself for at least many people.

Past reluctance to move a significant proportion of work to a home rather than office base for occupations where this is feasible — and where feasible, made all the more so because of the communications technologies that now exist — was predicated on the psychological desirability of human contact and its positive effects on productivity. The technologies of communication, under the pressure of necessity in lockdown and movement-limitation measures during COVID-19, rapidly advanced: Zoom, Teams and other platforms have replaced Skype as flexible, multifunctional channels for achieving much, even if not quite all, of what in-person contact offers. Cost considerations alone will cement the transfer from in-person to electronic contact in many cases: compare transporting a number of people physically by air to a meeting point in a distant city to convening a Zoom meeting of the same group.

There is a ramification of implications from this last point. To mention one: higher education (assuming equivalent impacts will be less in primary and secondary education) had to learn quickly how to adopt and adapt online delivery of courses. For laboratory and practice-based courses the inability to have on-site, in-person sessions was a major handicap; for the humanities and social sciences the challenge was less, and indeed in some respects suggested new ways to enhance student outcomes. One salient benefit was that recorded material could be accessed by students at any time of their choosing and repeatedly, leaving real-time contact — whether by Zoom or in person — to deeper exploration of the material thus already accessed.

Some students liked being able to attend lectures and seminars from their bedrooms, others missed the social contact that is a significant part of the university experience. But cost considerations, despite the resistance of universities which are highly conservative institutions, will inevitably drive delivery of higher education into cyberspace; this will eventually prove to be one of the pandemic's more significant consequences. For consider: to set up a new university from scratch, the standard model in the past has been to purchase hundreds of acres of greenfield sites and on them build lecture halls, libraries, halls of residence, laboratories and recreational facilities, and hire numerous faculty and administrative staff. Today and going forward, a new university can consist of iPads and tablets for students, a central administration commissioning content from freelance faculty and disseminating it on internet platforms, and online seminars. COVID-19 was a proof of concept for this model, and despite the rush to return to 'business as usual' as the current generation of students and faculty understand it, the great arbiter of financial considerations will doubtless have the last say.

In past pandemics almost everyone, apart from the small minority of nobles and clerics at the apex of society, was what today would be called a 'key worker' — transporting loads, clearing garbage, growing and harvesting food, cutting down trees, making shoes and clothing, burying the dead, doing the daily drudge work that keeps a society and its economy going. In COVID-19 essential services were maintained by low-paid workers in menial occupations, the vital nature of their various roles recognised if not rewarded in concrete-enough terms. Among the measures of preparation for likely forthcoming pandemics, accordingly, one is ensuring that 'key worker' roles are not taken for granted, but properly primed, organised and compensated.

The main point that emerges from comparing past pandemics to COVID-19, however, is that the big game changer is science, across the entire range from communications technologies to the genetic, biochemical and medical advances of recent decades which have resulted in opportunities for monitoring disease outbreaks, identifying pathogens, immunising against them, and treating them more effectively if immunisation fails or is only partly successful. In the century separating the Spanish Flu and COVID-19, the difference is dramatic. In the absence of the kind of resources available now, the Spanish Flu pandemic was devastating: a third of the world's then population of 1.5 billion was infected, and somewhere between 30 and

100 million died. The principal countermeasures were quarantine, personal hygiene, limitations on public gatherings and face masks. Medical knowledge in the Black Death and in outbreaks of infectious diseases right up to the 19th century had been premised on the ancient miasma theory of Galen, but even though the germ theory — of disease causation and transmission by pathogenic microorganisms — had superseded it, there was still no effective means to respond. These means now exist: future pandemics might resemble past pandemics in respect of changes in certain aspects of social behaviour and practice, but even though rates of morbidity and mortality will still be distressing to sufferers and those who care about them, there is reason to think that the scale of mayhem witnessed in past pandemics will, in relative terms, be more containable because of the transformative effect of scientific advances.

Chapter

10

Grey Rhino, Black Swan or Dragon King? The COVID-19 Pandemic in Historical Perspective

By Niall Ferguson

Summary

Since the completion and publication of *Doom: The Politics of Catastrophe* in the spring of 2021, we have learned several important things about the COVID-19 pandemic. Firstly, naïve attempts to blame responsibility for excess mortality on populist leaders lost whatever credibility they had. Second, the pandemic mortality exceeded most expectations, despite the speedy development of vaccines with high efficacy. Third, non-pharmaceutical interventions colloquially known as lockdowns succumbed to diminishing returns, most obviously in China. Fourth, the fiscal and monetary measures taken to offset the economic impact of lockdowns — which were comparable with those of a world war — turned out to be more inflationary than most economists foresaw. Fifth, as in previous times of plague, there was not only popular unrest but also war, the effect of which was to exacerbate the inflationary problem. Finally, it has become clear that the pandemic itself exacerbated global trends towards social, political and geopolitical instability that predated 2020.

I

It was one of the most memorable crossed wires of the Cold War. Asked in 1971 by Henry Kissinger for his opinion on the consequences of the French Revolution, the Chinese premier Zhou Enlai replied that it was "too early to say". That sounded profound — an expression of the Chinese ability to think long term, in centuries rather than the weeks preferred by Western statesmen. In fact, as the American diplomat Chas Freeman revealed in 2011, Zhou thought Kissinger was referring to the student protests of 1968, not the revolution of 1789 [1].

Is it too early to say what the consequences of the COVID-19 pandemic have been? One might argue that an historian should wait until an event is over before writing about it. But who is to say when a pandemic is over? The bubonic plague struck London repeatedly between 1348 and 1665. Influenza was a serial killer in the 20th century; it was never truly over. At the time of writing (September 2022), the disease is responsible for many fewer deaths per day (around 1,200) than at its peak in January 2021 (around 15,000). But it would be a foolish epidemiologist who ruled out the possibility of new variants in the future that might unleash new waves of infection, illness and death. We may have tired of the COVID-19 pandemic and yearn to return to "normal life", like children on a long car journey who soon after departure begin asking, "Are we nearly there yet?" But it seems increasingly probable that SARS-CoV-2 will become endemic and that we shall be playing the public health equivalent of Whac-a-Mole against new variants of the virus for years to come. In his most recent novel, *Termination Shock*, Neal Stephenson casually throws in a reference to "COVID-19, COVID-23, and COVID-27". If that is the future, the time to start addressing what went wrong in 2020 is now.

The general theory of disaster developed in my book *Doom: The Politics of Catastrophe* [2] can be simplified as follows. First, disasters are inherently unpredictable; they lie in the realm of uncertainty, not calculable risk. Attempts to foretell them almost always fail, though occasionally a Cassandra gets lucky. Some calamities may be discernible long before they strike: so-called grey rhinos [3]. And yet even these are perceived as black swans when they strike [4]. It is almost impossible to know at the outset which calamities will prove to be dragon kings [5] — defined here as disasters with historical consequences disproportionate to their death tolls. Second, there is no clear-cut dichotomy between natural and man-made disasters: excess mortality is almost always a function of human agency — hence "the politics of catastrophe", which is the best explanation for why the same virus had such different impacts around the world. Third, the crucial point of failure in most disasters is generally not at the top, but somewhere further down the chain of command (Richard Feynman's always unavailable "Mr Kingsbury"[a] at NASA [6]), though inept leadership can always make a bad situation even worse. Fourth, contagions of the body caused by pathogens often interact disruptively with contagions of the mind, in rather the same way that victory in war requires the destruction of both the enemy's materiel and his morale. Finally, because we cannot predict disasters, it is better to be generally paranoid than it is to be bureaucratically prepared for the wrong contingency. Rapidity of reaction to early warnings is the key to resilience, if not to anti-fragility, and — as Taiwan's COVID outbreak in May 2021 illustrated — it is easy to be a victim of one's own success if it leads to complacency.

Why did so many Western countries fail so badly to limit the spread of the new coronavirus SARS-CoV-2 in 2020, leading to some of the worst excess mortality we have seen since the 1950s? The success of Eastern countries such as Taiwan and South Korea — which successfully contained the initial spread of the virus while avoiding economically damaging lockdowns for more than a year — makes such a question legitimate. *Doom* argues that it is a mistake to lay all the blame for the Western democracies' failure on a few populist leaders, though their erratic leadership undoubtedly added something to the body count. What happened was a systemic failure of the public health bureaucracy — and this also appears to have happened in countries without populist leaders. There were pandemic preparedness plans; they simply did not work. Taiwan and South Korea owed their success in 2020 to a combination of rapidly scaled testing, contact tracing, and isolation of the potentially infected. In most Western countries, testing capacity was not built out swiftly enough; contact tracing was barely attempted; quarantines were not enforced; the vulnerable (especially in elderly care homes) were not protected but

---

[a] NASA's range safety officer, Lou Ullian, told Feynman "about the problems he had in trying to talk to the man in charge, Mr Kingsbury: he could get appointments with underlings, but he never could get through to Kingsbury and find out how NASA got its figure of 1 in 100,000" as the probability of the space shuttle's failing. Ullian's estimate was 1 in 100.

exposed. These were the costliest early mistakes in terms of loss of life, and it is not plausible that Donald Trump or Boris Johnson was personally to blame for any of them. Michael Lewis arrived at a similar assessment by a very different route in *The Premonition*. As one of his Cassandras notes, "Trump was a comorbidity" [7]. So was Johnson, if Dominic Cummings's account of the debacle in London is to be believed. The central point of Cummings's May 2021 testimony was not simply that the prime minister was "unfit for the job", but that the entire government failed: not just the elected politicians, but the civil servants and the public health experts — all fell "disastrously short of the standards that the public has a right to expect" [8].

If we tell ourselves that there would have been far less excess mortality with different presidents and prime ministers, we are therefore making a profound mistake. Ron Klain, Joe Biden's chief of staff, acknowledged in 2019 that, if the swine flu that struck the US in 2009 had been as deadly as COVID-19, President Barack Obama's administration would not have done much better: "We did every possible thing wrong. And…60 million Americans got H1N1 in that period of time. And it's just purely a fortuity that this isn't one of the great mass casualty events in American history. Had nothing to do with us doing anything right. Just had to do with luck" [9]. The events of 2021 — which saw 476,750 American deaths due to COVID, compared with 371,000 in 2020 — surely put an end to the naive argument that it was all Trump's fault.

The contrast with the Taiwanese experience seemed to me very striking. By coincidence, I had paid my first visit to Taipei in early January 2020, when stories of a mysterious new form of pneumonia in Wuhan were just beginning to circulate. Three things impressed me very much. First, the presidential election of January 11 went as smoothly as any election I have ever witnessed. Second, both public and private experts on cybersecurity and information warfare were well aware (and somewhat contemptuous) of attempts from the mainland to interfere in the democratic process. Third, Taiwan seemed to be applying computer science and software tools to public policy in a more creative way than any Western country, thanks in large measure to the influence of Audrey Tang, who had joined the government in August 2016. Justifiably mistrustful of assurances from Beijing that there was no human-to-human transmission of the Wuhan virus, the Taiwanese government applied Larry Brilliant's formula of "early detection, early action" with exceptional success. Throughout 2020, there were fewer than 800 cases of COVID-19 in Taiwan, and just seven deaths. This was partly because Taiwanese officials had learned the lessons of two previous coronavirus outbreaks, SARS and MERS. But there was more to Taiwan's success in 2020 than that. For example, a website was used to ration face masks when they were scarce. Had there been an outbreak in Taipei, officials had a plan to subdivide the city into neighbourhoods separated by *cordons sanitaires*. Schools remained open, albeit with elaborate and strictly enforced precautions.

II

Doom was written and copyedited by the end of October 2020. In the intervening two years there have been many important new developments, some of which I anticipated, some of which I did not. I was right to be optimistic about the Western vaccines, but even in my most confident moments I did not dare to hope for efficacy above 90 percent in the Pfizer-BioNTech and Moderna phase III trials. I also did not foresee how effectively Western governments that had so badly bungled containment of the virus would procure and distribute the vaccines. In these respects, I was too bearish.

On the other hand, I was much too bullish to think that total COVID-19 mortality would end up roughly where the Asian influenza pandemic of 1957–58 ended, killing around 0.04 percent of the world's population. The death toll is now significantly higher. As I write, at least 6.5 million people — 0.086 percent of the world's population — have died from COVID-19. However, this number is almost certainly an underestimate. The Institute for Health Metrics and Evaluation puts total deaths attributable to COVID at 17.6 million and projects a further 400,000 deaths by January 1, 2023. *The Economist* estimates excess mortality at between 16 million and 26.5 million, using a model that adjusts for undercounting of pandemic-related deaths in developing countries: a maximum of 0.35 percent of the global population. True, the relative death toll of 2020–21 will not match that of the 1918–19 Spanish influenza, which killed an estimated 1.7 percent of the world's population, five times higher than *The Economist's* maximum estimate. Moreover, allowing for the very different age profile of the victims and therefore the number of life-years lost, our pandemic still seems closer to that of 1957 than to that of 1918. (An even better analogy might be with the so-called Russian flu of 1889–90, which some modern researchers think may in fact have been caused by a coronavirus.) Nevertheless, I clearly underestimated the problems that would be posed by new variants capable of reinfecting people who had previously had earlier versions of the virus as well as of reducing vaccine efficacy, and therefore underestimated the death tolls of the later waves.

I also failed to foresee that governments in Asia that had been successful in suppressing the spread of the virus in 2020 would lag behind in vaccination precisely because of that success. Taiwan found itself poorly prepared for the arrival of new and more contagious variants of the virus and faced its first real outbreak in May–July 2021, when case numbers jumped above 7,000 and deaths rose above 700, at a time when only a tiny share of the population (0.1 percent) had received one vaccine dose and testing capacity had been allowed to shrink to dangerously low levels. A second and significantly larger wave swept the country in the summer of 2022 as the more transmissible Omicron variant of the virus spread around the world.

Another variable I misjudged in 2020 was how extraordinarily resilient anti-vaccine sentiment would be in the United States. In their resistance not only to vaccines but to lockdowns, masks, and other measures intended to protect public health, many Americans turned out to be social Darwinists, as sceptical of the intrusive and yet ineffective nanny state as Herbert Spencer was in his prime.

As the third anniversary of the outbreak of the pandemic approaches, it is possible to estimate which countries fared worst and which fared best. In terms of COVID-related mortality relative to population, the hardest-hit nations appear — with the exception of Peru — to have been in Central and Eastern Europe. Deaths per million of population exceeded 4,000 in Peru, Bulgaria, Bosnia, Hungary, Northern Macedonia, Montenegro, Georgia and Croatia. The United States ranked 16th in the world; the United Kingdom 29th. The least affected states — or those that counted the dead least accurately — were mostly in sub-Saharan Africa, with the notable exception of China, which claims a COVID mortality rate three orders of magnitude smaller than the United States (4 per million as compared with 3,230).

COVID was no disease for old men (or old women). In the United States, according to data from the Centers for Disease Control and Prevention, people aged 65 and older accounted for three quarters of COVID deaths, the under-25s for just 0.32 percent. As in the influenza pandemics of 1918 and 1957, the COVID pandemic came in waves. The remarkable thing in 2020–22 was the sustained excess mortality. The UK data point to two waves of excess mortality, with peaks in April 2020 and January 2021. British historical statistics help put COVID in perspective. 1918, 1940 and 1951 were more deadly than 2020 if one considers crude and age-adjusted mortality rates relative to the previous ten-year average, going back to 1847. It is not hard to see why there was high excess mortality in 1918 and 1940, but who now remembers the influenza epidemic of 1951? The *Daily Mail* described the winter of 1950–51 as "the worst winter for illness ever known" — a characteristic exaggeration [10]. On the same basis, the United States had experienced nothing so severe since 1918.

A striking feature of the COVID pandemic, compared with the influenza pandemics of the 20th century, is that the economic costs were out of all proportion to the public health impact. In late 2020 David Cutler and Lawrence Summers estimated that there would be 625,000 cumulative US deaths by the end of 2021 — an underestimate, as it turned out — but they put the total costs to the US economy at $16 trillion. This figure was "twice the total monetary outlay for all the wars the US has fought since September 11, 2001" and "approximately the estimate of damages (such as from decreased agricultural productivity and more frequent severe weather events) from 50 years of climate change." Including the approximate costs of premature death and debilitating physical or mental health impairment, the total economic impact was approximately 90 percent of GDP, far in excess of the estimated 3.5 percent contraction of output in 2020 [11].

COVID is a second-tier disaster by comparison with the world wars. Including all civilian deaths, World War II caused the premature deaths of 2.4 percent of the world's population, with the skew towards younger age groups because it was mostly young men who engaged in the deadliest forms of warfare. In terms of its fiscal and monetary impact, however, COVID *has* been like a world war. That is because, for the first time in history, we used lockdowns to combat contagion — because we could, thanks to modern communications technology — although the adaptive behaviour of people may have been just as important (perhaps even more so) in reducing economic activity at the height of the COVID panic in 2020. It is still too early to say if the benefits of lockdowns (a loose term that covered a wide range of policies to restrict mobility and sociability) delivered a public health benefit worth more than their cost [12]. However, it can be said with some confidence that those who argued for drastic non-pharmaceutical interventions in early 2020 almost certainly understated their indirect costs, including on physical and mental health [13].

III

What comes next? In a few sentences in his book *Apollo's Arrow*, my friend Nicholas Christakis asked if, in the wake of the pandemic we might find ourselves, like our great-grandparents and grandparents after the 1918–19 influenza pandemic, in the Roaring Twenties:

> The increased religiosity and reflection of the immediate and intermediate pandemic periods could give way to increased expressions of risk-taking, intemperance, or *joie de vivre* in the post-pandemic period. The great appeal of cities will be apparent once again. People will relentlessly seek opportunities for social mixing on a larger scale in sporting events, concerts, and political rallies. And after a serious epidemic, people often feel not only a renewed sense of purpose but a renewed sense of possibility. The 1920s brought the widespread use of the radio, jazz, the Harlem Renaissance, and women's suffrage [14].

To say the least, this was a rather flattering sketch of the 1920s — a decade as notable in the United States for its violent criminals as for its flappers and elsewhere mainly memorable for hyperinflation, hunger, Bolshevism, and fascism.

As noted above, it does not take much for a grey rhino — the easy-to-foresee kind of disaster — to become a suddenly surprising black swan when the disaster actually strikes. But it takes a lot for a black swan to become a dragon king, in my sense of an historic disaster the magnitude and significance of which exceed the raw body count. For that to happen, the initial spike of excess mortality needs to have economic, social, cultural, political, and geopolitical consequences that together constitute a cascade of disaster. It is already apparent that such a cascade is happening.

The public health consequences of the pandemic seem predictable. Recurrent outbreaks and new variants (which will continue to turn up so long as a large share of the world's population remains unvaccinated) may well necessitate our getting regular booster shots of vaccine, perhaps more frequently than every year; may force us to keep those irksome masks in our pockets and briefcases, if not on our faces; may oblige us periodically to resume taking tests and filling out online forms to enable us to get into offices and onto planes.

The economic consequences of the pandemic were still far from clear when *Doom* went to press. "Was it secular stagnation we had to fear," I asked, "or a return of inflation?" In February 2021 Larry Summers — the economist who had revived the idea of secular stagnation in 2014 — answered that question by warning that disproportionately large fiscal stimulus in the context of a relatively small output gap was likely to be inflationary in the United States (the discrepancy between policy response and slack was less pronounced elsewhere) [15]. This proved prescient. Eight months later, when the US consumer price inflation rate exceeded 6 percent, it was clear that a combination of excessively expansionary fiscal and monetary policy at a time of pandemic-related supply constraints had produced a jump in inflation that was more than "transitory", as the Federal Reserve had claimed, and that inflation expectations had slipped their anchor, rather as had happened in the second half of the 1960s. "Frankly we welcome slightly higher … inflation," the Federal Reserve chair Jerome Powell had said in January. "The kind of troubling inflation people like me grew up with seems unlikely in the domestic and global context we've been in for some time" [16]. That was imprudent.

As in the 1970s, geopolitical shocks added fuel to the inflationary fire. In the same way that the 1973 Arab-Israeli war in the Middle East drove prices upwards, so too did the Russian invasion of Ukraine exacerbate an existing inflation problem. True, it was unlikely that inflation would remain above 8 percent for long after the Federal Reserve embarked on raising interest rates and "quantitative tightening". But it was equally unlikely that inflation would return to around 2 percent by 2024. Moreover, tighter monetary policy would create its own financial and economic problems.

The political consequences of the pandemic were in some ways easier to foresee two years ago. Donald Trump lost a presidential election he would almost certainly have won had the pandemic not struck; Boris Johnson had been lucky to have his general election in December 2019, on the eve of destruction, but in the end he, too, fell victim to the pandemic when it became clear that he and other government officials had repeatedly broken their own lockdown rules. Even after all his sins of omission and commission of 2020, however, Trump still was not defeated in anything resembling a landslide.

The United States did not turn into the Weimar Republic, nor did a Second Civil War break out — though the events of January 6, when a motley mob of Trump supporters and votaries of the QAnon cult broke into the US Capitol, allowed those who had predicted such dire scenarios to claim vindication [17]. Polling shortly after the invasion of the Capitol revealed that a very large proportion of Republican voters (around 70 percent) did not accept that Trump had lost the election, but only a minority had a favourable view of those who had marauded through the nation's legislature [18].

Three things were clear about the events of January 6 by the time of their anniversary. First, it gave the big technology companies an opportunity to exclude Trump from social media and therefore the modern public square — a far more effective "coup" than the one personified by the ludicrous QAnon shaman. Second, Trump's near disappearance did not preclude a future political revival. Accusing the other side of having stolen the election, even after a foiled attempt to steal it himself, might turn out to be a viable strategy for victory in 2024, though it is hard to believe that by then a sufficient proportion of voters will care as much as Trump about what happened four years before. Third, Trump's conduct in trying to contest the election emboldened the incoming Democratic administration to the point of hubris. Biden had run and won as the "normalcy" candidate, the veteran of the middle ground. However, within a hundred days of his inauguration, his party's well-oiled policy machine brought forward a series of legislative measures — the American Rescue Plan, the American Jobs Plan, and the American Families Plan — with a combined cost of close to $6 trillion. There was heady talk of a "transformative" presidency, amplified by partisan media outlets, that seemed to overlook the Democrats' exceedingly slender majorities in both Senate and House, a stark contrast with the fat margins that had enabled Franklin Roosevelt and Lyndon Johnson to enact their ambitious domestic programs. It was not difficult to foresee the potential unintended consequences of Biden's early overreach: not only higher inflation, but also a surge of illegal border crossings from Mexico in response to the public repudiation of Trump's border wall, and a sustained increase in violent crime that dated back to the upheavals of the summer of 2020 precipitated by the killing of George Floyd [19].

Another underestimated political consequence of the pandemic was the increased exposure, during lockdowns, of many American parents to the content of their children's education at high school and college. The year 2021 was noteworthy for the surge of public aversion to the spread in schools and colleges of "wokeism" — the indoctrination of students with "critical race theory" and scientifically dubious ideas about sex and gender. At the same time, there was a growing awareness of the damage to young people's mental health caused by the disruption of education and social life during the pandemic [20].

The disaster of COVID has led to a wide variety of political responses around the world. Some democracies, such as the United States and Brazil, have threatened to come apart, as issues of public health — masks, lockdowns, vaccines, therapies — became politicised along party lines. Others, notably Germany and Italy, have achieved relatively smooth political transitions that at least temporarily diminished the influence of populists. Many authoritarian regimes have seized the opportunity presented by the pandemic to tighten their grip on their populations. But there has been a price to be paid in every case. China's "zero-COVID" policy became steadily more costly to sustain as variants of the virus grew more transmissible. In the spring of 2022, it brought the Chinese economy to a near standstill. The Russian government's crackdown on all political opposition has coincided with very high levels of pandemic mortality. Turkey's economy is beset by currency depreciation and double-digit inflation. Globally, there was already a trend toward greater social unrest — including demonstrations, riots, and strikes — in the years immediately before 2020 [21]. Perhaps future historians will see the pandemic as just part of an "avalanche" of instability that tipped a number of weak states (Afghanistan, Ethiopia, Lebanon) into the abyss [22].

Yet the most important consequence of the pandemic still seems to me to lie in the realm of geopolitics, not domestic politics. Cold War II, which had already commenced before the pandemic, showed every sign of continuing despite the change of administration in Washington, DC. As Biden's campaign had promised, his administration is in many ways tougher on China than its predecessor, broadening its criticisms of the Chinese Communist Party to include issues of democracy and human rights that never much interested Trump, and seeking to organise allies — notably Australia, India, Japan, as well as the United Kingdom — into something like a balancing coalition against China, an approach fundamentally different from Trump's indiscriminate protectionism and disdain for allies. No meeting of the Trump era had more of a Cold War atmosphere than Biden's Secretary of State Anthony Blinken's ill-tempered encounter with his Chinese opposite number, Yang Jiechi, at Anchorage in March 2021. Even the issue of climate change has become entangled with the Sino-American antagonism, as US representatives point out the preeminent role China has played in increasing greenhouse gas emissions over the past two decades. It is worth recollecting that, in its early phase, Cold War I produced a distinctly hot war in Korea. That a similar confrontation might escalate over Taiwan is one of the more obvious risks of the post-pandemic period. After all, Taiwan combines the qualities of Berlin, Cuba and the Persian Gulf in Cold War I: its status is contested, it is geographically very close to one of the superpowers and very far from the other, and it is to high-end semiconductors what Saudi Arabia is to crude oil. There are good reasons two greatest causes of excess mortality in history — pandemics and wars — often follow hard on each other's heels, when they do not march in lockstep. As it turned out, the first hot war of Cold War II broke out in February 2022, when Russia invaded Ukraine (for reasons that had nothing to do with COVID).

In Alan Bennett's play *The History Boys*, one of the provincial sixth-formers aspiring to an Oxford place is asked by a teacher to define history. "It's just one fucking thing after another," he replies [23]. To be more precise, history can sometimes seem like just one *disaster* after another. We cannot say with any certainty what form the next big disaster will take, or where it will strike. Nor can we foresee which societies will respond most effectively to it. Sometimes the disaster elicits a creative response, just as success tends to breed complacency.

In 1970, the year before Kissinger's meeting with Zhou, the first screen adaptation of Joseph Heller's novel *Catch-22* was released. Thanks to one of the screenwriters, the film includes a famous line that does not appear in the book: "Just because you're paranoid doesn't mean they aren't after you." I have come to see that this is the central message of *Doom*, too. Disasters of all shapes and sizes really *are* after us. The best way to prepare for them is not the kind of bureaucratic pseudo-preparation that cost so many lives throughout the Western world over the past two years. Nor does it help to impose a partisan slant on each disaster that strikes. Rather, we must try to cultivate the kind of general paranoia that Heller's World War II airmen felt. So long as we accept that success in averting disaster is rarely rewarded, we can at least attempt to do better the next time disaster strikes.

References

[1] McGregor, R (2011, June 10). Zhou's cryptic caution lost in translation. *Financial Times*. https://delanceyplace.com/view-archives.php?p=1711.

[2] Ferguson, N (2021). *Doom: The Politics of Catastrophe*. Penguin.

[3] Wucker, M (2016). *The Gray Rhino: How to Recognize and Act on the Obvious Dangers We Ignore*. Macmillan.

[4] Taleb, NN (2007). *The Black Swan: The Impact of the Highly Improbable*. Penguin/Allen Lane.

[5] Sornette, D (2009). Dragon kings, black swans and the prediction of crises. *Swiss Finance Institute Research Paper Series 09*, 36. http://ssrn.com/abstract=1470006.

[6] Feynman, R (1988). *What Do You Care What Other People Think?: Further Adventures of a Curious Character*. WW Norton.

[7] Lewis, M (2021). *The Premonition: A Pandemic Story*. WW Norton.

[8] Dominic Cummings: Thousands died needlessly after Covid mistakes (2021, May 26). *BBC News*. https://www.bbc.com/news/uk-politics-57253578.

[9] Kessler, G (2021, October 15). In context: what Biden aide Ron Klain said about the swine flu. *Washington Post*. https://www.washingtonpost.com/politics/2020/10/15/context-what-biden-aide-ron-klain-said-about-swine-flu/.

[10] 'Worst Winter' for illness (1951, January 19). *Daily Mail*.

[11] Cutler, DM & Summers, LH (2020). The COVID-19 pandemic and the $16 trillion virus. *JAMA*, **324**(15), 1495–1496.

[12] For a controversial first effort at a cost-benefit analysis, see Herby, J, Jonung, L & Hanke, SH (2022). A literature review and meta-analysis of the effects of lockdowns on COVID-19 mortality. *Studies in Applied Economics*, 200.

[13] Ferguson, N, *et al.* (2020, March 16). Report 9: Impact of non-pharmaceutical interventions (NPIs) to reduce COVID-19 mortality and healthcare demand. *Imperial College COVID-19 Response Team*. https://spiral.imperial.ac.uk:8443/handle/10044/1/77482.

[14] Christakis, N (2020). *Apollo's Arrow: The Profound and Enduring Impact of the Coronavirus on the Way We Live*. Little, Brown Spark.

[15] Summers, LH (2021, February 4). The Biden stimulus is admirably ambitious. But it brings some big risks, too. *Washington Post*. https://www.washingtonpost.com/opinions/2021/02/04/larry-summers-biden-covid-stimulus/.

[16] Jay Powell says 'We have not won this yet,' as Fed holds rates steady (2021, January 27). *Financial Times*. https://www.ft.com/content/3f860e2b-8173-4e3a-a9c1-fc9a8ac8939d.

[17] Serwer, A (2021, January 12). The Capitol rioters weren't 'low class'. *The Atlantic*. https://www.theatlantic.com/ideas/archive/2021/01/thoroughly-respectable-rioters/617644/; Phillips, MM (2021, January 10). One Trump fan's descent into the U.S. Capitol mob. *Wall Street Journal*. https://www.wsj.com/articles/one-trump-fans-descent-into-the-u-s-capitol-mob-11610311660; Pape, RA & Ruby, K (2021, February 2). The Capitol rioters

aren't like other extremists. *The Atlantic.* https://www.theatlantic.com/ideas/archive/2021/02/the-capitol-rioters-arent-like-other-extremists/617895/; Frankel, TC (2021, February 10). A majority of the people arrested for Capitol riot had a history of financial trouble. *Washington Post.* https://www.washingtonpost.com/business/2021/02/10/capitol-insurrectionists-jenna-ryan-financial-problems/.

[18] PBS NewsHour/Marist Poll (2021, January 7). *Marist College.* http://maristpoll.marist.edu/wp-content/uploads/2021/01/PBS-NewsHour_Marist-Poll_USA-NOS-and-Tables_202101081001.pdf#page=3.

[19] See my contribution to "The First Ninety-Nine Days" (2021, April 28). *Persuasion.* https://www.persuasion.community/p/the-first-99-days.

[20] Thompson, D (2022, April 11). Why American teens are so sad. *The Atlantic.* https://www.theatlantic.com/newsletters/archive/2022/04/american-teens-sadness-depression-anxiety/629524/.

[21] Global Peace Index 2021 (2021, June). *Institute for Economics and Peace.* https://www.visionofhumanity.org/resources/. See also Hadzi-Vaskov, M, Pienknagura, S & Ricci, LA (2021, May 7). The macroeconomic impact of social unrest. *International Monetary Fund Working Paper No. 2021/135.* https://www.imf.org/en/Publications/WP/Issues/2021/05/07/The-Macroeconomic-Impact-of-Social-Unrest-50338.

[22] For the concept of a "conflict avalanche", see Lee, ED, *et al.* (2020). Scaling theory of armed conflict avalanches. *Physical Review E,* **102,** 042312.

[23] Bennett, A (2006). *The History Boys.* Farrar, Straus and Giroux.

https://doi.org/10.1142/9789811262821_0011

Chapter

11

Evaluating COVID-19 in the Context of Global Catastrophic Risk

By Tom Hobson, Lara Mani, Catherine Rhodes, and Lalitha Sundaram

Summary

Overall, whether or not COVID-19 fits with particular definitions of global catastrophic risk (GCR), it provides a case from which researchers, policy makers and practitioners can learn and improve their understanding of how GCRs and responses to them might play out. Likewise, scholarship from the field of existential and GCR studies, and from global catastrophic biological risk (GCBR) studies in particular, can help inform broader understanding of the pandemic.

Introduction

GCR is a concept that has had frequent use within the existential risk research community. At a basic level, a distinction can be drawn with existential risks being of a scale that can threaten the survival of humanity as a whole (or civilisational collapse from which we cannot recover our current state of societal development), and GCRs being of a scale that threatens a substantial proportion of the global population.

At a more detailed level, there is at present no agreed definition of a GCR. Most definitions relate to global death tolls in the millions or billions [1–3], though some look further to catastrophic impacts in terms of economic loss or suffering. Among these definitions, COVID-19's impact might reach the lower end of the scale but would not count as a GCR under definitions that focus on scenarios that kill hundreds of millions or billions of people.

Nonetheless, there are important reasons for evaluating COVID-19 in this context, which motivate this chapter. The rarity of GCR events means that research must rely on smaller catastrophes for empirical evidence to inform understanding of higher-impact scenarios. In general, the field of existential and GCR studies is moving towards greater focus on the systemic nature of such risks, cascading and cumulative impacts, and COVID-19 helps the field to explore these dimensions:

> analysis of potentially catastrophic events that were averted or mitigated might bring to light some of the approaches we can use to respond to or prepare for a global catastrophic biological event... With each consequential outbreak, new parameters are set and studied...and the response communities, local, national and regional, have additional and iterative tools to deal with the next outbreak [4].

Efforts to evaluate GCRs necessitate interdisciplinary working, which is reflected in the perspectives presented in this chapter, unified by an interest in how GCRs are framed and the implications this has for their evaluation, as well as how evaluating COVID-19 in this context can enhance our understanding of GCRs. In particular, we examine: implications of COVID-19 for understanding which events have GCBR potential; lessons for and from communication during global catastrophes; how COVID-19 demonstrates the systemic nature and policy challenge of responding to GCBRs; and how a co-benefits approach, aimed at improving governance and simultaneously enhancing resilience to GCRs, might be a useful way of meeting this challenge.

Global Catastrophic Biological Risks

Work at the intersection of biosecurity, global health security and GCR studies expanded significantly around five years ago, and there is now a sub-field of GCBRs linking experts from these areas. Early conceptual work on GCBRs included commentaries on a working definition provided by the Johns Hopkins Center for Health Security in a 2017 special issue of *Global*

Health Security. Useful insights for evaluating COVID-19 in this context can be found in that work, particularly where it extends beyond a sole focus on fatalities. The working definition:

> those events in which biological agents — whether naturally emerging or reemerging, deliberately created and released, or laboratory engineered and escaped — could lead to sudden, extraordinary, widespread disaster beyond the collective capability of national and international governments and the private sector to control. If unchecked, GCBRs would lead to great suffering, loss of life, and sustained damage to national governments, international relationships, economies, societal stability, or global security [5].

Other contributors noted that "While a sudden attack may be more likely to overwhelm controls, a global catastrophic biological event need not occur suddenly or even all at once: Multiple concordant or sequential events, each of which might have lower individual impact, might together produce a catastrophe..." [6].

Whether or not COVID-19 is viewed as having reached the lower end of the scale of GCBRs, it provides probably the best case study we have about how such events may play out, the challenges we are likely to face in addressing them, and the value of preparedness. It emphasises the importance of dimensions beyond fatality rates, such as the disruption of 'societal stability' [7], in achieving a fuller understanding of the catastrophic impacts of biological risks. Contributors to the special issue also point to the importance of understanding that a biological risk that might not constitute a GCR taken in isolation, when combined with other events may significantly contribute to global catastrophes, and is likely to increase our vulnerability to a range of GCRs for many years, if not decades to come [8, 9].

It is also clear that the shape and speed of our response matters for whether an outbreak might become a GCBR. Here we can learn not just from the areas that might be improved in how we responded to COVID-19, but also from the pathways through which it could have been much worse. As we may not be able to accurately assess the severity of an event at the point necessary for timely interventions, we may need to respond to more biological risks as potential GCBRs, and this points towards placing high value on measures and systems that improve resilience and reduce vulnerability to a range of biological risks. This would not be limited to the perhaps more obvious health system capacities, surveillance, and countermeasures, *etc.*, but would extend to broader societal and economic shifts that enhance resilience, such as addressing poverty and inequality as significant drivers of severe outcomes.

Incorporating Chronic Disease Threats into Understanding of GCBRs

Absent from most GCBR discussions is understanding whether and how chronic disease threats could have GCBR potential. Evaluating COVID-19 in the context of GCRs prompts additional consideration of outbreaks that combine acute and chronic components.

We focus here on communicable chronic diseases, although we recognise that some definitions tend to limit the term to non-communicable disease. A broadly useful working definition, enabling us to draw out features of relevance in the context of COVID-19 and GCRs, emphasises long duration of symptoms or sequelae (not necessarily continuous in nature) and uses morbidity as well as mortality in assessing GCBR potential, recognising that disease need not be fatal to be greatly harmful.

There are previous examples of significant long-term sequelae from infectious disease outbreaks. Poliomyelitis is an obvious example, but so are outbreaks more readily associated with the COVID-19 pandemic, such as the 'Russian Influenza' outbreak of 1889–92 [10] in which "The official end of the pandemic, therefore, did not mean the end of illness but was merely the prelude to a *longue durée* of baffling sequelae" [11]. Thus, though we are still in the early stages of understanding COVID-19 sequelae, it is clearly necessary to consider its impacts in both the long and short term [12], and to add this to our evaluation of potential GCBRs.

In our analysis of chronic diseases and GCBRs, several disease-centric characteristics emerged relevant to evaluating the global experience of COVID-19: communicability, detectability, ease of diagnosis, availability/accessibility of control measures, duration, physiological effects, and care requirements. As with COVID-19, any asymptomatically transmissible disease is difficult to contain without robust screening programmes. This was starkly the case with polio, where quarantine proved virtually ineffective because, although not spread through airborne routes like COVID-19, it is nevertheless very communicable via the faecal-oral route, and has a long pre-clinical phase of asymptomatic infection. Conversely, a long lag between infection and the onset of chronic symptoms could allow time for the development and deployment of countermeasures. The quantity of care required can also present a more significant impact in chronic conditions. However, health metrics such as QALYs and DALYs [13] rarely incorporate externality-based measures such as loss of carers' income, let alone broader societal impacts, which are particularly significant in the GCBR context.

In evaluating chronic diseases as potential GCRs, one useful framework outlines three key dimensions: critical systems, global spread mechanisms, and prevention/mitigation failures [14]. Global spread is a prime consideration for infectious diseases; these also affect and are affected by numerous critical systems. Health-related disasters can drastically reduce the labour force, which affects all aspects of societal functioning, not least systems tasked with prevention and mitigation. These impacts are likely to be longer lasting where there is a significant chronic burden, and can set a multi-generational trap where, especially in contexts of poverty, development goals are not achieved because of these lasting effects.

HIV/AIDS and Long COVID

The example of HIV/AIDS is instructive here, presenting several hallmarks of GCBRs [15], of chronic disease and comparisons to COVID-19. In the early 1980s, otherwise healthy gay men in large US cities exhibited symptoms of conditions usually related to old age or immunocompromise: the first hints that 'something was amiss'. While we now recognise these as signs of late-stage HIV infection, the lag had important implications. As noted by UNAIDS: "The nature of the virus meant that the extent and impact of AIDS, unlike other pandemics...remained hidden.... This 'silent' epidemic made it easier for leaders to remain silent in their response" [16]. Looking back at the characteristics that are likely to be important in assessing GCBR potential, difficulty in detection (a diverse 'constellation' of clinical symptoms) and long latency are particularly significant, the latter strongly contributing to rapid global spread.

Since it was first recognised, HIV/AIDS has resulted in approximately 36.3 million deaths globally. Neither these, nor the socioeconomic impacts, have been equally distributed. Two-thirds of people living with HIV/AIDS are in Sub-Saharan Africa; this region also accounts for almost half of HIV/AIDS deaths [17]. While these fatality figures would exclude HIV/AIDS from some definitions of GCR, if we include aspects related to 'significant shifts in human trajectory', impact on international relations and global stability, a different conclusion can be reached, one that has significance for how we evaluate COVID-19 in this context, and how we assess future threats. Several major studies pointed to the severe impacts of the epidemic in Sub-Saharan Africa. In 1999, a World Bank Report warned against inaction in the face of the growing epidemic: "The resulting social decay and breakdown will threaten socioeconomic development for decades to come" [18]. An International Labor Organization working paper warned that "the epidemic affects social and economic life in ways we have never seen before" through impacts across all sectors, including essential services. Over the longer term the report noted, "The epidemic is eroding the capacity for development through its effects on labour supplies, saving rates, national security and social cohesion" [19].

HIV/AIDS in Sub-Saharan Africa resulted in severe disturbances to numerous societal and economic "critical systems" [2]. While the most severe impacts occurred within a particular geographic region, this does not mean that they were not 'globally catastrophic'; the contributions made by Africa to global development will have been profoundly shaped by this, having significant impacts on humanity as a whole. Especially with diseases with chronic components, the nature of these impacts will shift over time. For HIV/AIDS, the 'chronicity' of the disease means that "adherence challenges, episodes of serious illness, transaction and opportunity costs related to lifelong treatment, and the need for continued investment of public resources to fund treatment programmes will all put serious and sustained pressure on communities and states alike" [20]. When considering COVID-19 and future GCBRs, we should be aware that disturbances of critical systems are more likely to transform than disappear when outbreaks move beyond an acute phase.

There are also several features relating to prevention and mitigation failures that exhibit parallels and important differences in global responses to HIV/AIDS and COVID-19. Early in the HIV/AIDS epidemic, developed countries saw fervent attempts at containment and mitigation, and the development of treatments: in some ways, this is paralleled by the exceptional measures that were instituted in several countries in 2020–21 but perhaps more so by the gamble on COVID-19 vaccine investment. When, in Western countries, a generalised HIV/AIDS epidemic failed to materialise, popular attention decreased and "much of the sense of urgency among the general public was lost" [21]. It is difficult not to see the parallel here with post-lockdown Western societies where a sense that the pandemic is over or has become endemic seems to prevail [22].

Despite the lack of Western attention to HIV/AIDS in the late 1990s, rates of infection were rising to catastrophic levels elsewhere and not being recognised, because of poor data, cultural ignorance, and outright denial [16]. The associated delay was compounded by internal politics, poverty and global inequality in the response. There seems to have been a similar dwindling of Western attention to global COVID-19, but instead of (largely) successful prevention campaigns and the development of anti-retrovirals, in the case of HIV/AIDS, this seems to be due to development of vaccines — or rather, the accessibility of vaccines — in wealthy countries. Unequal distribution of vaccines for COVID-19 is a likely indicator of the overall way in which global disease impacts (including those of Long COVID) will be unequally distributed. Further parallels emerge in the functioning of intellectual property rights during health emergencies [23, 24].

The impacts of these early decisions are already apparent, with UNDP estimating that had vaccination rates been more equal, "low-income countries' GDP would have increased by $16.27 billion" in 2021 [25]. The additional benefits that might have occurred had those funds been available for 'other development priorities' are difficult to calculate but should not be ignored in our learning for future GCBRs. Evaluating the effects of Long COVID will present additional challenges, with data even more scarce from low- and middle-income countries than for acute infections, and capacities to participate in associated research, as well as establishing healthcare responses, extremely limited [26, 27].

Co-Benefit Approaches and The Policy Challenge of GCBRs

As the above discussion concerning the parallels between Long COVID and HIV/AIDS begins to uncover, there are significant interactions between the parallel crises of inequality/inequity, global health and the preparedness and resilience of societies to GCBRs. Evaluating COVID-19 can aid our understanding of these interactions and connected policy challenges. Here we focus on challenges related to the provision and maintenance of robust governance systems for scientific research, and challenges related to addressing inequality, poverty and injustice, and how lessons drawn can serve efforts to prevent, mitigate or recover from global catastrophes.

In seeking to build societal resilience to GCRs, the concept of co-benefits (as developed by Sundaram *et al.* [28]) supports arguments that investment in these types of social and political goods will likely play a strong role in effective governmental preparedness efforts. Certain characteristics of biological hazards make this approach particularly appropriate for GCBRs. Indeed, it may be the case that potentially catastrophic biological risks are more effectively addressed through such measures — that enhance capacities for governance and societal resilience — than through alternative measures that mobilise the language and practices of national security and prohibitions. The latter often seek to insure against the risks of biological research or harmful pathogens without additionally addressing social, political and governance contexts that drive these risks or render societies vulnerable to their occurrence.

Alongside the definition of GCBRs as events where a biological agent could lead "extraordinary, widespread disaster beyond the collective capability of national and international governments" and ultimately to "great suffering, loss of life, and sustained damage to national governments, international relationships, economies, societal stability, or global security" [5], such events may catalyse an acute crisis or precipitate the emergence of new, ongoing social and geopolitical conditions. These events may be the result of agents that are "naturally emerging or reemerging, deliberately created and released, or laboratory engineered and escaped". Below we highlight some of the ways by which each of these may be addressed.

Biological Security, Responsible Science and Good Governance

Life sciences research is diffuse, varied and rapidly advancing. It takes place in a wide range of contexts and contributes, in many settings, to significant advances in human health, knowledge and well-being. The problem of ensuring the 'goods' of biological research while proscribing the potential harms is frequently characterised by the notion of Dual Use. The broader problems of ensuring against accidental release or deliberate misuse of biological agents in laboratory settings are captured in the parallel concepts of biological safety and biological security. While these issues are subject to various treaties and regulatory frameworks, the challenges posed by contemporary advances in, and proliferation of, biological research capabilities have reinvigorated debates about how education, normative regimes, collaboration and good governance can supplement more traditional regulatory frameworks. The nature of this challenge was summarised in recent evidence submitted to the *Biosecurity Strategy Review* [29]:

> Biological technology capabilities are expanding rapidly and international regimes governing biological research date back several decades. The convergent and frenetic nature of biotechnology advances raise significant proliferation concerns — and presents incremental as well as more fundamental challenges to the existing global biological weapon control regime.

And the WHO's draft *Global Guidance Framework for the Responsible Use of the Life Sciences* [30] notes that effective responses will require the enhancement, and deeper embedding of, biosecurity education at all levels:

> A chronic and fundamental challenge is that practising scientists, technologists, and other managers and funders of scientific research and technology development lack a basic awareness that their work — which is predominantly undertaken to advance knowledge and tools to improve health, economies and societies — could be conducted or misused in ways that result in health and security risks to the public. There is also a lack of incentives for these groups to identify and mitigate such risks.

Such education efforts can enable safer and more responsible scientific practices in the present, while simultaneously mitigating against the types of error or misuse that could cause biological catastrophe. Enhancing capabilities for early and ongoing biotechnology assessment would perform the function of improving the operational effectiveness of governance regimes, whilst also facilitating early recognition of potential extreme risks posed by technological advances.

With technology assessment and horizon scanning recognised as persistent challenges for mitigating biological risks, enhancing cooperation and coordination of this type, and fostering strong normative regimes relating to responsible practice are likely to be effective measures. This straightforwardly constitutes a co-benefit: enhancing contemporary governance and building trust in its systems, whilst also providing enhanced capacity for prevention, detection, and mitigation of potentially catastrophic biological events.

With preparedness activities in the UK criticised as overly focused on pandemic influenza scenarios, there is clearly value in shifting focus away from the potential occurrence of discrete, individual crises and towards developing robust governance, enhancing cooperation, and improving practices. This argument was explored by Maas *et al.* [31] who argued for a focus on "vulnerability and exposure rather than existential hazards" and drew attention towards "latent structural vulnerabilities in our technological systems and in our societal arrangements [which] may increase our susceptibility to existential hazards".

COVID-19 has increased attention to biological risks from all sources, including those resulting from laboratory accidents or deliberate misuse. This increases the need for effective governance arrangements and processes for identifying and addressing techno-scientific vulnerabilities, efforts which, carefully designed and implemented, will produce co-benefits for responsible scientific practice and for mitigation of extreme risks.

Pandemics, Public Health and Inequality

The COVID-19 pandemic (as well as prior experiences) clearly demonstrate how inequality and inequity exacerbated many of the problems of the resulting public health crisis. A number of accounts describe how the structural effects of poverty and inequality served to either drive high levels of infection during the COVID-19 pandemic, or significantly hampered efforts to respond to the outbreak in lower- and middle-income countries. Even within wealthy countries, there is substantial evidence of differentiated health outcomes and mortality rates, as well as impacts of second-order socioeconomic costs, between different socioeconomic groups [32]. Issues such as crowding, poor sanitation access and inadequate social safety nets were all reported to account for higher mortality and morbidity [33]. One of the clearest areas of global inequality in the COVID-19 response has been in the distribution of vaccines [34], which has been compounded by the handling of intellectual property right arrangements for COVID-19 vaccines, diagnostics and treatments, during what is clearly a global health emergency [35]. This has had impacts in terms of excess deaths and severe economic impacts. The IMF noted in 2021 that as long as such disparities in access exist, "the inequalities in health and economic outcomes will increase, driving further divergences across two blocs of countries" [36]; and UNDP has estimated a loss of over $16 billion from low-income countries' GDP in 2021 compared to the situation had there been more equitable vaccination rates [37].

Efforts to address these issues — including efforts to improve healthcare and vaccine equity between countries, policies and funding to increase access to sanitation and improve local health services, and overall efforts towards more fairly distributing the costs and benefits of our present socioeconomic contexts — will have powerful co-benefits: serving to create a safer and more just world now, and better preparing societies to prevent, mitigate and respond to GCRs.

Co-Benefits, Intrinsic Risks and Structural Vulnerabilities

Maintaining robust governance mechanisms, increasing cooperation and redressing injustice and inequality can serve to foster a better world today whilst also reducing the likelihood of severe harm from global catastrophes that may occur in the future. Improvements in these areas will not only bring benefits for addressing biological risks, but for the range of global challenges that we face, many of which will rely on the same systems and structures for societal resilience. This is likely to represent a course of action that is more cost effective and adaptive than a narrower focus on discrete, individual potential crises. For researchers and those with responsibility for management of GCRs, it both responds to the growing understanding of the systemic nature of risks and vulnerabilities [2], and engages with the positive narratives facilitated by the concept of co-benefits.

This approach allows us to engage in a meaningful way with the systemic or even intrinsic nature of many of the drivers of risk, and vulnerabilities to it, that are features of our contemporary social and political contexts. The notion of co-benefits argues that undertaking the basic work of enhancing governance capabilities, and addressing societal inequalities, will necessarily also enhance our preparedness for and resilience to GCBRs.

Effective Communications for GCBRs

Communication remains an important tool in preparing and alerting our societies to potential unfolding GCBRs. COVID-19 provided us with an insight into how well national governments and international organisations were able to communicate the risks of an unfolding disease outbreak, to varying degrees of success. Several studies have examined and analysed various aspects of the global communication response (*e.g.*, [38, 39]), so we focus here on some key successes from COVID-19 and other crises that can inform how we consider communication about future GCBRs and other GCRs.

Pandemic and Disease Outbreak Simulation Exercises

To stress test national response mechanisms to unfolding crises, simulation exercises are often used with stakeholders to assess the ability of national systems to cope with such scenarios and to identify areas for improvement in national and international responses. Scenario exercises have been widely used for this purpose in the face of a biosecurity threat. In 2018, the WHO ran pandemic preparedness simulation exercises with 40 countries to stress test their pandemic response [40]. Similarly, the Johns Hopkins Center for Health Security have been running highly immersive, high-cost, realistic scenarios for natural pandemics (*e.g.*, exercise Event 201 simulating a novel coronavirus outbreak prior to the COVID-19 pandemic) and even for deliberate release of pathogens in terrorist attacks (*e.g.*, exercise Dark Winter simulating the spread of smallpox and Clade X simulating a novel pathogen) [41–43].

Despite the sophistication of some of these exercises, the recommendations and suggested improvements identified during the scenarios are often ignored by those tasked with preparing for such events. A key example was the report findings from Operation Cygnus run by Public Health England in 2016, warning that the UK's health system was unprepared for the dealing with mass patients from a respiratory disease outbreak and that Personal Protective Equipment (PPE) stockpiles were insufficient [44]. Despite this warning prior to COVID-19, the UK's health service became quickly overwhelmed and lacked necessary equipment such as ventilators and appropriate PPE. Scenario exercises can assist stakeholders in their preparations for potential evolving

GCBRs, and indeed for other GCRs (scenarios are also widely used for simulations of other GCRs including asteroid strikes, nuclear winter scenarios and natural disasters). However, the COVID-19 pandemic revealed that despite many countries participating in simulation exercises, many of whom were considered to be well prepared for the next global pandemic, preparedness could have been enhanced by the adoption of recommendations from such exercises. Therefore, prioritisation must be given to implementation of the findings and recommendations of such simulations in order to strengthen national response to future pandemics, and simulation exercises should be routinely used to stress test resilience strategies in the face of GCRs.

Global Early Warning Systems and Alert Levels

The use of alert levels to communicate risk in an unfolding crisis is best demonstrated within the field of disaster risk [45–47]. Alert levels can be used to demonstrate how serious a risk is posed to individuals with the risk level often depicted using a traffic light colour system, with green as low risk and red as high risk. Although not commonly used during the COVID-19 crisis, alert levels used by the New Zealand government to portray the risks posed to the public, and the prevention actions to be taken [48], proved a successful example of their potential use for unfolding biosecurity threats. Development of a global early warning alert level system, and associated structures to observe, set and monitor for GCBRs and biological threats could help minimise loss of life and reduce the social and economic impacts of such an event [49].

Improved Community Sensitisation to Biosecurity Risks

A basic step that can also be taken to reduce the spread of disease outbreaks is use of simple education and awareness campaigns. Commonly employed in regions of the world where disease outbreaks are a frequent occurrence, such as the Caribbean for dengue fever, and West Africa for Ebola outbreaks, raising awareness of communities to identify signs and symptoms of diseases and sharing of methods to reduce risk, such as through basic hygiene and safe water storage, can influence risk-reducing behaviours, making people more likely to take preventive actions [50]. In such regions, sensitisation of communities towards the risks posed by disease outbreaks is often achieved through the influence of cultural products and expansive education programmes. A similar approach could be used on a larger scale to prepare the global community for future bio-risks, particularly in the aftermath of COVID-19 where risk awareness amongst the general population remains high. Starting by simply building basic healthcare measures for reducing the transmission of disease into school curricula is a straightforward step in advancing this, particularly as school-age children are known to pass such information on to their parents [51]. Even during a time of uncertainty during a disease outbreak, public awareness campaigns can prove successful in increased adoption of preparedness measures and empowering communities to build their resilience, thus lessening the impacts [52].

Inclusivity and Equity in Communication

One of the key aspects that remains important in a GCR event, no matter the source of the risk, whether it be a natural pandemic or an asteroid strike, is to ensure the equity and accessibility of information and neutrality in messaging. Neglect of communities based on language barriers, accessibility needs or cultural differences, and the use of derogatory terms relating to the origins of the virus were evident throughout the COVID-19 pandemic. This led to numerous instances of racial abuse and marginalisation [53], and the blaming of localised outbreaks on minority groups excluded from key information briefs [54]. Without ensuring communications messages are made as inclusive and equitable as possible, dealing with a potential disease outbreak and unfolding GCBR will become very difficult, and the impacts could be much graver [55]. The COVID-19 pandemic clearly demonstrated the need for careful consideration around how we communicate during a future unfolding pandemic, particularly around the importance of maintaining public trust through the concise communication of uncertainty, empowering or solutions-based messages, and through the rapid dispelling of mis- and dis-information.

Forward Look to a Future Pandemic

Several major groups are now working to use the current window of opportunity and increased attention COVID-19 has brought to reiterate the message that we are not only unprepared for events at this scale, but also for the more severe events we may face in future — GCBRs. These concerns span not only naturally occurring pandemics, but also those that might result from accidental releases or deliberate attacks. Whether these activities will be more successful and sustained than similar messages around pandemic preparedness prior to COVID-19 is uncertain, and may struggle for prioritisation among a range of other urgent global challenges. This points to a need to focus on actions that can increase our resilience to a range of catastrophic risks, so that cycles of panic and neglect can be avoided.

In each dimension that we have considered, efforts to address global inequalities are key to substantive progress in preparing for and responding to global catastrophes. A few specific examples (among many) in which there would ideally be substantive progress in advance of a future pandemic include:

- Planning and mechanisms in place for robust data collection and analysis globally, and extending beyond short-term outcomes, to more accurately reflect societal impacts [12].
- Attention to accessibility and inclusivity in communication, with mechanisms in place to prevent or mitigate misinformation and stigmatisation of certain groups or countries.
- Extensive and sustained capacity building in health systems and workforces, and for safe and secure life sciences research.
- Systems for more equitable distribution of diagnostics, treatments and vaccines, that can withstand countries' tendencies towards actions that serve narrowly conceived 'national interest', rather than prioritising global pandemic response.

Conclusion

When evaluating COVID-19 in the context of GCRs, the important question is not whether COVID-19 constitutes a GCR, but what it can teach us in regard to such extreme risks and approaches to their prevention, management and mitigation. These are areas of high uncertainty, and so while we must also be wary of the tendency to 'fight the last war', the value of information we can get from any 'not quite' GCRs or near misses is high. We will also have opportunities for further learning over the next few decades as we will be able to assess the extent to which an event of this type affects our vulnerability to other catastrophes, and whether it will prompt advanced actions for resilience to risks of this scale.

References

[1] Bostrom, N & Cirkovic, MM (2008). *Global Catastrophic Risks*. Oxford University Press.

[2] Avin, S, Wintle, BC, Weitzdörfer, J, Ó hÉigeartaigh, SS, Sutherland, WJ & Rees, MJ (2018). Classifying global catastrophic risks. *Futures*, **102**, 20–26.

[3] Turchin, A & Denkenberger, D (2018). Global catastrophic and existential risks communication scale. *Futures*, **102**, 27–38.

[4] Connell, ND (2017). The challenge of global catastrophic biological risks. *Health Security*, **15**(4), 345–346.

[5] Schoch-Spana, M, Cicero, A, Adalja, A, Gronvall, G, Kirk Sell, T, Meyer, D, Nuzzo, JB, Ravi, S, Shearer, MP, Toner, E, Watson, C, Watson, M & Inglesby, T (2017). Global catastrophic biological risks: toward a working definition. *Health Security*, **15**(4), 323–328.

[6] Palmer, MJ, Tiu, BC, Weissenbach, AS & Relman, DA (2017). On defining global catastrophic biological risks. *Health Security*, **15**(4), 347–348.

[7] George, D (2017). How should we define global catastrophic biological risks? *Health Security*, **15**(4), 339–340.

[8] Yassif, J (2017). Reducing global catastrophic biological risks. *Health Security*, **15**(4), 329–330.

[9] Cameron, EE (2017). Emerging and converging global catastrophic biological risks. *Health Security*, **15**(4), 337–338.

[10] Which some have speculated was a Coronavirus pandemic, *e.g.*, Brüssow, H & Brüssow, L (2021). Clinical evidence that the pandemic from 1889 to 1891 commonly called the Russian flu might have been an earlier coronavirus pandemic. *Microbial Biotechnology*, **14**(5), 1860–1870.

[11] Honigsbaum, M & Krishnan, L (2020). Taking pandemic sequelae seriously: from the Russian influenza to COVID-19 long-haulers. *The Lancet*, **396**(10260), 1389–1391.

[12] Alwan, NA (2021). The teachings of Long COVID. *Communications Medicine*, **1**(1), 15.

[13] Sassi, F (2006). Calculating QALYs, comparing QALY and DALY calculations. *Health Policy and Planning*, **21**(5), 402–408.

[14] Avin, S, Wintle, BC, Weitzdörfer, J, Ó hÉigeartaigh, SS, Sutherland, WJ & Rees, MJ (2018). Classifying global catastrophic risks. *Futures*, **102**, 20–26.

[15] Schoch-Spana, M, Cicero, A, Adalja, A, Gronvall, G, Kirk Sell, T, Meyer, D, Nuzzo, JB, Ravi, S, Shearer, MP, Toner, E, Watson, C, Watson, M & Inglesby, T (2017). Global catastrophic biological risks: toward a working definition. *Health Security*, **15**(4), 323–328.

[16] Knight, L (2008). UNAIDS: The first ten years, 1996–2006. *Joint United Nations Programme on AIDS*. https://data.unaids.org/pub/report/2008/jc1579_first_10_years_en.pdf.

[17] Fact sheet — Latest global and regional statistics on the status of the AIDS epidemic (n.d.). *UNAIDS*. https://www.unaids.org/sites/default/files/media_asset/UNAIDS_FactSheet_en.pdf.

[18] Intensifying action against HIV/AIDS in Africa: responding to a development crisis (1999). *The World Bank*. https://documents1.worldbank.org/curated/en/412891468192857140/pdf/Intensifying-action-against-HIV-AIDS-in-Africa-responding-to-a-development-crisis.pdf.

[19] Cohen, D (2002). Human capital and the HIV epidemic in sub-Saharan Africa. *ILO Working Papers*. https://www.ilo.org/public/libdoc/ilo/2002/102B09_378_engl.pdf.

[20] Colvin, CJ (2011). HIV/AIDS, chronic diseases and globalisation. *Globalization and Health*, **7**(1), 31.

[21] Smith, JH & Whiteside, A (2010). The history of AIDS exceptionalism. *Journal of the International AIDS Society*, **13**(1), 47.

[22] This phenomenon is apparent as: "A period of high social and public attention accompanied by bitter debates is inevitably followed by a phase of *fatigue and declining interest in the issue.*" — described in Rosenbrock, R, Dubois-Arber, F, Moers, M, Pinell, P, Schaeffer, D & Setbon, M (2000). The normalization of AIDS in Western European countries. *Social Science & Medicine*, **50**(11), 1607–1629.

[23] Hoen, ET, Berger, J, Calmy, A & Moon, S (2011). Driving a decade of change: HIV/AIDS, patents and access to medicines for all. *Journal of the International AIDS Society*, **14**(1), 15.

[24] Lack of a real IP waiver on COVID-19 tools is a disappointing failure for people (2022, June 17). *Médecins Sans Frontières (MSF) International*. https://www.msf.org/lack-real-ip-waiver-covid-19-tools-disappointing-failure-people.

[25] Impact of vaccine inequity on economic recovery 2022 (2022, February). *UNDP Data Futures Platform*. https://data.undp.org/vaccine-equity-archive/impact-of-vaccine-inequity-on-economic-recovery-2022/.

[26] Michelen, M, Manoharan, L, Elkheir, N, Cheng, V, Dagens, A, Hastie, C, O'Hara, M, Suett, J, Dahmash, D, Bugaeva, P, Rigby, I, Munblit, D, Harriss, E, Burls, A, Foote, C, Scott, J, Carson, G, Olliaro, P, Sigfrid, L & Stavropoulou, C (2021). Characterising long COVID: a living systematic review. *BMJ Global Health*, **6**(9), e005427.

[27] Adeloye, D, *et al.* (2021). The long-term sequelae of COVID-19: an international consensus on research priorities for patients with pre-existing and new-onset airways disease. *The Lancet Respiratory Medicine*, **9**(12), 1467–1478.

[28] Sundaram, L, Maas, MM & Beard, SJ (2022). Seven questions for existential risk studies. *SSRN*. http://dx.doi.org/10.2139/ssrn.4118618.

[29] Hobson, T, *et al.* (2022). Submission of evidence to the Cabinet Office enquiry on the biological security strategy. *Cabinet Office*. https://doi.org/10.17863/CAM.82937.

[30] Global guidance framework for the responsible use of the life sciences (2022, February 22). *WHO*. https://www.who.int/publications/i/item/WHO-SCI-RFH-2022.01.

[31] Liu, HY, Lauta, KC & Maas, MM (2018). Governing boring apocalypses: A new typology of existential vulnerabilities and exposures for existential risk research. *Futures*, **102**, 6–19.

[32] Oronce, CIA, Scannell, CA, Kawachi, I *et al.* (2020). Association between state-level income inequality and COVID-19 cases and mortality. *Journal of Internal Medicine,* **35,** 2791–2793; Sepulveda, ER & Brooker, AS (2021). Income inequality and COVID-19 mortality: age-stratified analysis of 22 OECD countries. *SSM — Population Health,* **16,** 100904.; Patel, JA, Nielsen, F, Badiani, AA, Assi, S, Unadkat, VA, Patel, B, Ravindrane, R & Wardle, H (2020). Poverty, inequality and COVID-19: the forgotten vulnerable. *Public Health,* **183,** 110–111.

[33] Cardoso, E, Silva, M, De Albuquerque Felix Junior, FE, De Carvalho, SV, De Carvalho, A, Vijaykumar, N & Frances, C (2020). Characterizing the impact of social inequality on COVID-19 propagation in developing countries. *IEEE Access: Practical Innovations, Open Solutions,* **8,** 172563–172580.

[34] WHO vaccine dashboard (2022, June). *WHO.* https://covid19.who.int/?mapFilter= vaccinations.

[35] Countries obstructing COVID-19 patent waiver must allow negotiations to start (2021, March 9). *Medicins Sans Frontiers, Press Release.* https://www.msf.org/ countries-obstructing-covid-19-patent-waiver-must-allow-negotiations.

[36] Chapter 1 Global Prospects and Policies (2021). In *World Economic Outlook, October 2021.* International Monetary Fund.

[37] Kaizer, F (2022, March 28). UN analysis shows link between lack of vaccine equity and widening poverty gap. *UN Health News.* https://news.un.org/en/story/2022/03/1114762.

[38] Hyland-Wood, B, Gardner, J, Leask, J & Ecker, UKH (2021). Toward effective government communication strategies in the era of COVID-19. *Humanities and Social Sciences Communications,* **8**(1), 1–11.

[39] Varghese, NE, Sabat, I, Neumann-Böhme, S, Schreyögg, J, Stargardt, T, Torbica, A, Exel, J van, Barros, PP & Brouwer, W (2021). Risk communication during COVID-19: A descriptive study on familiarity with, adherence to and trust in the WHO preventive measures. *PLOS ONE,* **16**(4), e0250872.

[40] Simulation exercise puts global pandemic readiness to the test (2018, December 3). *WHO.* https://www.who.int/news-room/feature-stories/detail/simulation-exercise-puts-global-pandemic-readiness-to-the-test.

[41] O'Toole, T, Michael, M & Inglesby, TV (2002). Shining light on "Dark Winter". *Clinical Infectious Diseases,* **34**(7), 972–983.

[42] Public-private cooperation for pandemic preparedness and response (n.d.). *Johns Hopkins Center for Health Security.* https://www.centerforhealthsecurity.org/event201/ recommendations.html.

[43] Clade X Exercise: Improving policy to prepare for severe pandemics (n.d.). *The Johns Hopkins Center for Health Security.* https://www.centerforhealthsecurity.org/our-work/ events/2018_clade_x_exercise/pdfs/Clade-X-executive-summary-document.pdf.

[44] Exercise Cygnus report: Tier one command post exercise pandemic influenza (2017). *Public Health England.* https://assets.publishing.service.gov.uk/government/uploads/ system/uploads/attachment_data/file/927770/exercise-cygnus-report.pdf.

[45] Fearnley, CJ (2022). Volcanic Hazards Warnings: Effective Communications of. In Tilling, RI (Ed.), *Complexity in Tsunamis, Volcanoes, and their Hazards*, pp. 717–742. Springer.

[46] Potter, SH, Jolly, GE, Neall, VE, Johnston, DM & Scott, BJ (2014). Communicating the status of volcanic activity: revising New Zealand's volcanic alert level system. *Journal of Applied Volcanology*, 3(1), 13.

[47] Zschau, J & Küppers, A (2003). *Early Warning Systems for Natural Disaster Reduction*. Springer.

[48] History of the COVID-19 Protection Framework (traffic lights) (n.d.). *Unite against COVID-19*. https://covid19.govt.nz/traffic-lights/.

[49] Fearnley, CJ & Dixon, D (2020). Editorial: Early warning systems for pandemics: lessons learned from natural hazards. *International Journal of Disaster Risk Reduction*, 49, 101674.

[50] Wang, M & Fang, H (2020). The effect of health education on knowledge and behavior toward respiratory infectious diseases among students in Gansu, China: a quasi-natural experiment. *BMC Public Health*, 20(1), 681.

[51] Ronan, KR & Johnston, DM (2003). Hazards education for youth: a quasi-experimental investigation. *Risk Analysis: An Official Publication of the Society for Risk Analysis*, 23(5), 1009–1020.

[52] Awareness campaigns help prevent against COVID-19 in Afghanistan (2020, June 28). *World Bank*. https://www.worldbank.org/en/news/feature/2020/06/28/awareness-campaigns-help-prevent-against-covid-19-in-afghanistan.

[53] Coronavirus: Ukraine protesters attack buses carrying China evacuees (2020, February 21). *BBC News*. https://www.bbc.com/news/world-europe-51581805.

[54] Muslim Women Australia: Responding to COVID-19 (n.d.). *Muslim Women Australia*. https://mwa.org.au/latest-articles/muslim-women-australia-responding-to-covid-19/.

[55] Reddy, BV & Gupta, A (2020). Importance of effective communication during COVID-19 infodemic. *Journal of Family Medicine and Primary Care*, 9(8), 3793–3796.

Index

www.ingramcontent.com/pod-product-compliance
Lightning Source LLC
Chambersburg PA
CBHW050600190326
41458CB00007B/2122